Case presentations and MCQs for the MRCG

£17.24
m

Commissioning Editor: Ellen Green
Project Editor: Ninette Premdas
Project Controller: Fiona Young
Designer: Erik Bigland

Case presentations and MCQs for the MRCGP

Antonio A T Chuh

MRCP (UK) MRCP (Ire) MRCGP FRACGP MFM DCH DCCH DPDerm Dip G-U Med

Honorary Assistant Professor in Family Medicine
Department of Medicine
The University of Hong Kong

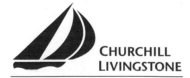

CHURCHILL
LIVINGSTONE

EDINBURGH LONDON NEW YORK PHILADELPHIA ST LOUIS SYDNEY
TORONTO 2000

CHURCHILL LIVINGSTONE
An imprint of Harcourt Publishers Limited

© Harcourt Publishers Limited 2000

🖢 is a registered trademark of Harcourt Publishers
Limited

The right of Dr A Chuh to be identified as author of this
work has been asserted by him in accordance with the
Copyright, Designs and Patents Act 1988.

First published 2000
 Reprinted 2000

ISBN 0 443 064199

British Library Cataloguing in Publication Data
A catalogue record for this book is available from the British
Library.

Library of Congress Cataloging in Publication Data
A catalog record for this book is available from the Library
of Congress.

Medical knowledge is constantly changing. As new
information becomes available, changes in treatment,
procedures, equipment and the use of drugs become
necessary. The author and the publishers have, as far as it
is possible, taken care to ensure that the information given
in this text is accurate and up to date. However, readers
are strongly advised to confirm that the information,
especially with regard to drug usage, complies with the
latest legislation and standards of practice.

The
publisher's
policy is to use
**paper manufactured
from sustainable forests**

Printed in China

PREFACE

This book is written for candidates sitting the MRCGP or other postgraduate examinations in general practice such as MICGP, FRACGP, MRNZCGP or MMed (Family Medicine). Medical students undergoing their general practice clerkship might also find the book useful.

Fifty clinical scenarios are presented as short essay questions. They encompass most of the problems commonly encountered in practice and in examinations. Constructs, or summaries, are suggested for each answer. Candidates can thus develop the habit of tackling each question systematically. Four MCQ papers are given, including extended matching questions. These closely simulate the actual examination.

I wish to thank Churchill Livingstone for their invaluable assistance in this project.

A A T Chuh

CONTENTS

INTRODUCTION

The MRCGP is a credit accumulation examination. The four modules are:

- Paper 1 (short answers, examiner-marked)
- Paper 2 (MCQ, machine-marked)
- Assessment of consulting skills (either video-recording or simulated surgery if video-recording is not feasible)
- Oral examination.

All modules may be taken at the same diet of the examination or at different diets. The order of taking the modules is entirely flexible: oral examination may be taken before the papers. All modules must be passed within 3 years, and a maximum of three attempts is allowed for each module. Otherwise, the entire examination must be repeated.

Candidates eligible to take the examination are independent practitioners or being trained to be so. Thus candidates in the UK must have either the Certificate of Prescribed or Equivalent Experience issued by the JCPTGP or their number on the Principals List of a Health Authority. GP registrars can take the examination at any time during their training, but can only take up Membership of the College once vocational training has been completed.

Overseas candidates must provide evidence of being an independent practitioner (eligible to practice unsupervised) in their country of residence. There is no specified period for them to be in active general practice after registration.

In addition, certificates of proficiency in cardiopulmonary resuscitation and child health surveillance are to be submitted before the examination. The submission of a log diary is not required.

Results for each module are now reported as Fail, Pass or Pass with Merit. If you achieve a Pass in all four modules within 3 years you earn a Pass in the whole examination, and, upon paying the Membership fees, Membership of the College. (For GP registrars, vocational training would still have to be completed.)

If you achieve a Pass with Merit in two modules with a Pass in the other two you earn an overall Pass with Merit. If you Pass four modules with Merit or Pass three modules with Merit and in the fourth acheive a Pass you attain an overall Pass with Distinction.

PAPER 1 (SHORT ANSWERS PAPER)

Candidates have to answer 12 or more questions in 3 hours; this means about 15 minutes for each question. Additional time to read source material for certain questions is provided in advance of the 3 hours.

There are four types of questions in the new Paper 1, which combines the former essay and critical reading papers:

(i) questions testing knowledge and interpretation of GP literature (*journal* questions)
(ii) questions testing interpretation of written material (*critical appraisal* questions)
(iii) questions testing theoretical knowledge and professional values (*clinical* and *situation* questions)
(iv) other questions (usually testing the wider perspectives of GP, e.g. socioeconomic, medicolegal, medicopolitical, ethical; these questions are usually not presented as a clinical case or practice situation).

Each question carries the same marks, and therefore the time spent on each should be roughly equal. Usually about 50% of the questions are clinical or practice situation questions, with two to three journal questions and two to three critical appraisal questions. There are usually only one or two questions from the fourth category.

Clinical and practice situation questions

These questions occupy about half of Paper 1. Their importance lies not only in their number but also in the fact that they are relatively easy to prepare well for. The preparation should be targeted at three areas:

- acquiring the core knowledge of common GP problems and situations
- learning to use appropriate *constructs* to different types of questions
- practising to use time effectively.

Although the College has in the past stressed that factual knowledge is mainly tested in the MCQ paper, much factual knowledge is also required to answer clinical and practice situation questions. A wide perspective has to be taken, and this must be built on core knowledge. Otherwise, the answer will appear 'hollow' and not substantiated with evidence.

As an example, consider a question on the goals of treatment for a girl with frequent episodic asthma. The candidate rightly turns to physical aspects first, mentioning 'To decrease the frequency of severe attacks' as a physical goal. However, a medical student or even a lay person can be expected to say that. As a postgraduate Membership level examination, more is expected. If the candidate can put down 'To decrease the frequency of severe and life-threatening attacks', so much the better. It then appears to the examiner that at least the candidate has read something about asthma.

A better candidate will then go on to outline a few points on the defining features of *severe attacks* and *life-threatening attacks*, quoting the newest guidelines of the British Thoracic Society.

Such core knowledge may be acquired using one of the several core textbooks on general practice. Reading large medical textbooks is to be discouraged. These should only be used as reference for this examination. Review articles in the *British Medical Journal (BMJ)* and *British Journal of General Practice (BJGP)* definitely help, and smaller *summary* texts (e.g. *ABC of...*, *Lecturer Notes in...*) should be read wisely and selectively.

Apart from acquiring a wide base of relevant core knowledge, the establishment of an appropriate *construct* in the answer is also important. Constructs come in many forms, e.g.

- aspects – physical, psychological, social, ethical
- prevention – primary, secondary, tertiary
- prevention – work to be done by the patient themself, by the family, by the GP and PHCT, by hospital specialists, by local health authorities, by the police, by social workers, by legislation, by the government
- secondary prevention (screening) – use Wilson and Jungner's criteria as a basic construct
- tertiary prevention – complications in terms of impairment, disability and handicap
- management – history, examination, investigations, treatment
- management – immediate management, short-term management, long-term plans

- management – managing the physical, psychological and social problems, managing the family as a whole (always ask: Who are the patients?)
- dealing with a controversial problem – list pros and cons of each alternative
- dealing with an emergency – ABC first, other immediate treatment, short-term measures, long-term management plan
- implications – implications to the physical and psychosocial health of the patient, to their work and hobbies, to the family, to the GP, to the PHCT, to the hospital, to the health authorities, to society
- implications – medical, psychological, social, financial, ethical and legal
- the audit cycle – standard setting, determining performance, comparing performance with standard, closing the audit loop.

A good construct sets out the answer in systematic and structured form. An answer with a not-so-good knowledge base usually appears much more informative when laid out in a structured form. It also guides the candidate to cover a wider perspective and think of more relevant points.

To be able to make the use of constructs second nature, take 30 clinical and practice situation questions and devise constructs for all of them without writing down the exact answers. Note that more than one construct may be used for any one question, and constructs may appear in compound forms, i.e. one inside another. Your constructs can then be compared with those of your colleagues.

In this book, the answers to the individual cases are presented mostly as short essays so as to preserve integrity of the concepts discussed. In the actual examination, however, short sentences can be used.

Lastly, you should have at least one opportunity of doing a mock examination paper under timed conditions. As most candidates will know something about most questions in this paper, the effective use of time right from the first question is essential.

Journal questions

Like the clinical and practice situation questions, you can obtain a high score in journal questions if you prepare well. Attending an examination course is of course helpful, but you really cannot escape from reading about 12–18 issues of *BJGP* and selective readings of several months' *BMJ*, *Doctor* and *General Practitioner (GP)*. A study group or a journal-club-ad-hoc is convenient, but not all candidates have such luxury.

When I took the MRCGP, I found that most of the major papers in *BJGP* can be summarised in 100 words. I did such for only 18 issues, which took me three nights. Before the examination I went through my summaries once and found this to be adequate for a comfortable pass.

Critical appraisal questions

For these questions, nothing can replace either a good study group or a short examination course. There are good books specifically in this area. However, the key to success is practice under examination conditions. Concepts not often covered in standard texts but which may come out are *yield, incremental yield, odds-ratio, relative risk* and *number needed to treat*.

Other questions – the fourth category

About 50% of the syllabus for these questions is centred around professional values and ethics. The hot topics are:

- alternative medicine
- autonomy and advocacy
- burnout
- clinical protocols
- complaints, protocol for in-house complaints procedure
- confidentiality
- consent to treatment
- continued education for GPs and the PHCT
- difficult patients
- evidence-based medicine
- fundholding
- GPs with poor performance/psychiatric problem/drug and alcohol abuse
- heartsink patients
- help-seeking behaviours
- housekeeping (awareness of one's own emotions)
- living wills, testamentary capacity and power of attorney
- patient presenting *the list* (a list of problems)
- practice computerisation
- reaccreditation
- relationship with specialists
- terminal care
- workplace safety.

Discussion of these topics can be found in issues of *BJGP*, *Doctor* or *GP*. This is a part of the examination in which participation in an examination course particularly helps.

Paper 2 (MCQ paper)

Paper 2 is mainly designed to test factual knowledge and its application. There are two sections. The first section contains questions of multiple true/false answers. A stem or statement is followed by up to six items. There can be up to 400 items in total.

The second section includes extended matching questions. A list of options is given, and a typical clinical scenario is to be matched to one of the options. To simulate the real diagnostic process, there are usually more options than scenario items, and one of the options can be the correct answer (usually diagnosis) to more than one scenario.

Questions of the single best answer type are also included in the second section. A statement or stem is followed by a number of items, only one of which is correct.

The second section may include up to 100 items.

To score well in this paper, a good knowledge base, good technique in answering MCQ questions and thorough understanding of common MCQ terms are needed. The knowledge can usually be acquired through preparation for Paper 1, i.e. via reading journals and short textbooks in the individual specialties. Reading a large internal medicine text is again *not* recommended. The choice of short textbooks is of individual preference, but emphasis should be placed in the specialties of medicine, surgery, OG, child health, psychiatry, dermatology, ophthalmology and ENT. A knowledge of basic statistics and epidemiology is also needed, but it is *not* advisable to read an individual text such as *An Introduction to Medical Statistics*.

5

Introduction

Negative marking was used in the past to discourage guessing. This is still being adopted in several other examinations. The disadvantage of such is that female candidates with a tendency to answer questions only if they are pretty sure of the answer are put at a disadvantage. The secret is that the more items answered, the higher the score is likely to be. This has been proved with theoretical models and experimental trials. The logical advice now is to *answer all questions with a best guess approach.* To avoid such negative discrimination of female candidates (who as a group do better in the whole examination), negative marking has now been abandoned in the MRCGP examination and thus all items should be attempted.

Several MCQ wordings warrant special attention:

Pathognomonic and *Diagnostic* mean that the presence of the feature (e.g. sign, symptom, phenomenon) is adequate to allow a diagnosis to be made: *the feature cannot occur in other conditions.*

Pathognomonic and *Diagnostic* do not give any indications of the prevalence of the feature in the disease. For example, erythema marginatum is pathognomonic of rheumatic fever. It cannot occur in other diseases (although it can be confused with erythema multiforme). However, less than 50% of all cases of rheumatic fever have erythema marginatum.

Characteristic means that the feature is highly suggestive of a disease but can occur in other conditions.

Characteristic again does not give any indication of the prevalence of the feature in the disease. For example, Köbner phenomenon is characteristic of lichen planus. However, less than 50% of patients with lichen planus display this phenomenon, and other conditions such as psoriasis and viral warts also show this phenomenon.

In the vast majority literally means that the feature is present in most patients with the disease, and gives an indication of the prevalence of the feature (usually taken as more than 90%). It does not give any indication of the occurrence of the feature in other diseases. In other words, it does not imply whether the feature is pathognomonic, diagnostic or characteristic.

For example, cafe-au-lait spots are present in the vast majority of patients with neurofibromatosis-1 (NF-1). The absence of such patches does not exclude NF-1, provided that the diagnostic criteria is met. Cafe-au-lait spots can occur in other conditions, such as tuberous sclerosis, McCune–Albright syndrome, Fanconi's anaemia, Russell–Silver dwarfism and indeed in normal individuals (although their number, size, margin and shape may differ in different conditions).

(In the MRCGP regulations, *Pathognomonic, Diagnostic, Characteristic* and *In the vast majority* are defined as exactly the same: implying that a feature would occur in at least 90% of cases. This is slightly different from general clinical usage. Upon discussion with several GP tutors, it is generally agreed that candidates are better advised to stick to the generally accepted definitions.)

Typical, Frequently, Significantly, Commonly and *In a substantial majority* are defined in the MRCGP regulations as implying that a feature would occur in at least 60% of cases. Thus these terms give an indication of the prevalence of the feature but do not imply their occurrence in other diseases. However, in general, if a condition is exclusively found in a disease, the terms *pathognomonic* or *diagnostic* will be used.

Definitions of other terms are given in the regulations and are not repeated here.

CONSULTING SKILLS ASSESSMENT

As the *Handbook on Consulting Skills Assessment* is very detailed and more than
90–95% candidates pass this segment at their first attempt, no additional advice is
given here. The candidates who do fail are likely not to have paid sufficient
attention to visual cues of the patients or not to have completed most parts of the
tasks of the consultations in many of their recordings.

This segment does pose special problems for overseas candidates whose
patients cannot speak English. It may be better to accumulate a videotape of
consultations gradually (over several weeks), asking only those patients who do
speak English to participate, than to opt for the simulated surgery alternative, in
which even more factors are beyond the control of the candidates.

ORAL EXAMINATION

Two consecutive orals each lasting 20 minutes will be given, with a break of 5
minutes between the two. The competence of the candidate is judged by four
examiners.

The oral examination in the MRCGP is highly structured. About five questions
will be asked in each 20 minute session, giving an average of 4 minutes per
question. The areas covered in the questions are *care of patients, working with
colleagues, social role of general practice* and *the doctor's personal responsibilities*.
Examiners will try their best to cover each of these areas in turn. Questions will be
individually marked. Each session is also individually graded by each examiner.
After the second oral the four examiners then meet to decide whether the
candidate deserves a Pass with Merit, a Pass or a Fail.

It is highly controversial whether candidates should guess from the question the
area that the examiner is aiming at. Some GP tutors and candidates think that
accurate identification of the area(s) being marked is a trainable technique.
However, if that identification is wrong, the question will be badly scored. Moreover,
more than one area will be covered by any one question.

My advice therefore is that unless the question is very specifically asking for one
of the target areas, one should not guess. In fact, before taking the orals myself, I
did my best to *forget* the areas being tested. This does not mean that the answers
are going to be unstructured. On the contrary, when a new question is asked, you
should spend about 2 seconds forming a skeleton in your mind, and then follow
your skeleton to give a well structured answer.

The processes involved in answering oral questions are therefore similar to the
short answer paper: the use of constructs is highly desirable. The examiner will
perceive your answer as systematic, you will always know what areas you are
going to cover, and the construct will lead to more and more points to cover as you
sail along. Moreover, provided that the construct you have chosen is an appropriate
one, it will almost always cover the target area in the minds of the examiners.

It must be emphasised that constructs are *not* a must for every question; for
simple straightforward questions requiring one or two simple sentences to answer,
the obsessive use of constructs is actually irritating to the examiners. However,
such questions are usually follow-up questions. For new questions covering new
target areas, the use of constructs is strongly advisable.

CONCLUSION

The MRCGP is not difficult, as more than 70–75% of all candidates usually passed in previous diets (the pass rates for the new format cannot be expressed so simply because of multiple modules). However, certain groups (candidates not born in the UK and Eire, those who have not received graduate education in the UK and Eire, those not residing in the UK and Eire, those not vocationally trained in the UK and Eire) may need to make a special effort, as their pass rates are generally lower.

The MRCGP is one of the few postgraduate medical examinations demonstrated to have high validity and reliability. It is a serious examination and deserves respect. With adequate preparation and practice, most candidates will find that this hurdle is fair and easily overcome.

Best of luck in the MRCGP and in other future examinations.

A A T Chuh

LIST OF ABBREVIATIONS

ABC	airway, breathing and circulation	**INR**	international normalised ratio
ABPM	ambulatory blood pressure measurement	**IUCD**	intrauterine contraceptive device
AC	air conduction	**IUGR**	intrauterine growth retardation
AIDS	acquired immunodeficiency syndrome	**IVDU**	intravenous drug user
BC	bone conduction	**KOH**	potassium hydroxide
b.i.d.	twice a day	**LDL**	low density lipoprotein
BMI	body mass index	**LOS**	lower oesophageal sphincter
BP	blood pressure		
BTS	British Thoracic Society	**MAOI**	monoamine oxidase inhibitor
CBC	complete blood count		
CIN	cervical intraepithelial neoplasia	**MMR**	measles, mumps and rubella
CIS	carcinoma in-situ	**MRI**	magnetic resonance imaging
CLO	*Campylobacter*-like organism	**NIDDM**	non-insulin-dependent diabetes mellitus
CNS	central nervous system		
COC	combined oral contraceptive	**NSAID**	non-steroidal anti-inflammatory drug
COPD	chronic obstructive pulmonary disease	**OG**	obstetrics and gynaecology
CT	computerised tomography	**OPD**	outpatient department
CVA	cerebrovascular accident	**PCR**	polymerase chain reaction
CVS	cardiovascular system	**PFR**	peak flow rate
DBP	diastolic blood pressure	**PHCT**	primary health care team
DM	diabetes mellitus	**PID**	pelvic inflammatory disease
ECG	electrocardiogram	**PMS**	premenstrual syndrome
ENT	ear, nose and throat	**p.r.n.**	as required
ESR	erythrocyte sedimentary rate	**QCA**	quadricyclic antidepressant
		q.i.d.	four times a day
GI	gastrointestinal	**RIMA**	reversible inhibitor of monoamine oxidase
GP	general practitioner		
GUM	genito-urinary medicine	**SARI**	serotonin-2 antagonist/reuptake inhibitor
HAV IgG	hepatitis A immunoglobulin G		
HbA$_1$	glycosylated haemoglobin 1	**SBP**	systolic blood pressure
HbA$_{1c}$	glycosylated haemoglobin 1c	**SLE**	systemic lupus erythematosus
HBeAg	hepatitis B envelope antigen		
HC	head circumference	**SNRI**	serotonin noradrenalin reuptake inhibitor
HCG	human chorionic gonadotrophin		
		SSRI	selective serotonin reuptake inhibitor
HDL	high density lipoprotein		
Hib	*Haemophilus influenza* type b	**STD**	sexually transmitted disease
HIV	human immunodeficiency virus	**T$_3$**	triiodothyroine
		T$_4$	thyroxin-4
HMG-CoA	hydroxymethyl glutaryl coenzyme A	**TCA**	tricyclic antidepressant
		t.d.s.	three times a day
HPV	human papillomavirus	**T/M**	trichomonas and monilia
HRT	hormone replacement therapy	**TSH**	thyroid stimulating hormone
		UTI	urinary tract infection
HSV	herpes simplex virus	**VDRL**	Venereal Disease Research Laboratory
HT	hypertension		
IBS	irritable bowel syndrome	**VLDL**	very low density lipoprotein

Mrs Eden, aged 28 years, is planning for her first pregnancy. She has DM and asthma and is on insulin, regular inhaled steroid and inhaled bronchodilator on a p.r.n. basis. Discuss your role as her GP before, during and after her pregnancy.

CONSTRUCT

Pre-pregnancy

- Aspects
  - physical
  - psychological
  - social
- Areas of concern:
  - effects of DM on mother
  - effects of DM on fetus
  - effects of pregnancy on DM
  - effects of asthma on pregnancy
  - effects of pregnancy on asthma.

Antenatal

- Physical
- Psychological
- Social.

Intrapartum

Postpartum

- Physical
- Psychological
- Social.

ANSWER

Pre-pregnancy

- Possible effects of asthma and DM on the pregnancy, and effects of pregnancy on the diseases, should be discussed so that the couple might make an informed choice beforehand and understand the importance of good control of the diseases and close monitoring of the mother and fetus.
- Summary of the effects:
  - effects of DM on the mother: urinary tract infection, candidiasis, gestational hypertension, polyhydramnios, preterm labour
  - effects of DM on the fetus: congenital abnormalities (transposition of great arteries, sacral agenesis, anal atresia), IUGR, respiratory distress, cerebral palsy, macrosomnia, brachial plexus injuries, unconjugated hyperbilirubinaemia, polycythaemia, hypocalcaemia, hypomagnesaemia
  - effects of pregnancy on the DM: poor control, need for increased insulin
  - effects of asthma on the pregnancy: IUGR if asthma poorly controlled, drug effects
  - effects of pregnancy on asthma: one-third of patients get better, one-third remain the same, one-third get worse.

- The control of asthma (symptoms, signs, effects on daily activities, PFR, drug compliance) and DM (home glucose monitoring, compliance, HbA_{1c}, microalbuminuria, complications) should be assessed.
- Psychological preparation for pregnancy and parenthood is essential.
- Psychological preparation for breastfeeding is best done before pregnancy.
- The couple should be seen together.
- Social support should be assessed; help from PHCT should be mobilised if needed.
- A close liaison with the respiratory physician and the endocrinologist is better established before the pregnancy.
- Problems should be anticipated, e.g. poor DM and asthma control, social and emotional difficulties.
- Counselling should be given for other areas of pre-pregnancy concern, including smoking, alcohol, nutrition, exercise, folic acid, etc.

Antenatal

- The care of pregnancies with potential complications is best delegated to the hospital obstetrician, as close maternal and fetus monitoring is essential.
- The GP should ensure that appointments in the antenatal, respiratory and endocrine clinics are properly arranged (best if on the same days) and punctually attended by Mrs Eden.
- The diet should be well regulated, and the dose of insulin gradually increased depending on blood glucose levels.
- Inhaled bronchodilators used p.r.n. are continued. Systemic steroids are avoided and inhaled steroids, though with minimal teratogenic potential, should be continued if indicated. Premature withdrawal of prophylactic inhaled steroids may lead to attacks, necessitating rescue courses of systemic steroids that are far less desirable.
- The possibility of postpartum depression is always best discussed antenatally, as psychological preparation is beneficial.

Intrapartum

- Early elective admission may be needed to optimise control of the DM and asthma before delivery.
- Caesarian section is performed for obstetric indications only.
- Glucose/insulin drip is given during delivery, with continuous fetal heart monitoring and fetal blood sampling if indicated.
- The baby is admitted to a special baby care unit after delivery if needed.

Postpartum

- The postpartum checkups may be performed by the GP (shared care) or the obstetrician.
- Postpartum complications, e.g. haemorrhage, fever, infections, depression, are attended to as usual.
- The insulin may be gradually decreased as needed.
- Both DM and asthma are not contraindications to breastfeeding, which should be encouraged within the first 2 hours after birth.
- Counselling for family planning and contraception is given.
- A Personal Child Health Record is given to Mrs Eden. The baby should attend checkups and receive immunisations as scheduled. Support from the PHCT should be available.

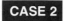

Elaine, aged 25 years, has carcinoma of the ovary with liver secondaries. The tumour showed little response after 1 year of chemotherapy. The gynaecologist suggested use of newer agents, with many adverse effects.

Elaine wanted to add life to her years (perhaps months) and not years to her life. She turned to nutritional and herbal therapies. She wanted you, as her GP, to monitor her cancer marker CA125 and arrange regular liver ultrasound to monitor the size of the secondaries, so that she might compare the effects of the two styles of therapy on the control of her tumour.

What problems can arise from her request?

CONSTRUCT

- Problems relating to the patient
- Problems relating to the GP
- Problems relating to the PHCT
- Problems relating to the practice
- Problems relating to the gynaecologist
- Ethical problems
- Medicolegal problems.

ANSWER

There can be many immediate and potential problems:

- doctor–patient relationship. If her request is refused, the doctor–patient relationship is adversely affected. This can have long-term effects on the future care and support.
- relationship with the gynaecologist. If her request is followed, the care will be transferred from the gynaecologist to the GP. The pride of the gynaecologist can be affected and he may see this transferral as his failure to help Elaine. Future liaison between the gynaecologist and the GP is affected.
- ability of the GP and the PHCT. Do the GP and PHCT have the necessary expertise to manage and support her? Elaine's condition can deteriorate anytime and terminal care, pain control and psychosocial support will have to be delivered by the GP and the PHCT.
- workload and emotional stress of the GP and the PHCT. The workload is obviously increased, especially if frequent home visits are necessary later. Caring for terminal patients may be emotionally rewarding for some health workers, but it is emotionally draining for most.
- continuity of care. The care is transferred from the gynaecologist to the GP and other alternative therapists. The care and support may not be smooth and continuous.
- attitude of the GP to alternative therapies. The GP may not believe in such therapies. However, he will inevitably be asked to comment on these by Elaine in the future. He may find it difficult to make constructive comments.
- conflicts with evidence-based medicine. Apart from the paucity of evidence for the beneficial effects of nutritional and herbal therapies in the control of malignancies, there is also no evidence that CA125 and liver ultrasound can be used to monitor the response to such treatment. Is it ethical for the GP to practise in this manner?
- collusion of anonymity. The healers will not be part of an integrated team and collusion of anonymity is bound to exist. Elaine might have to make decisions by herself. Will such decisions be informed choices? What happens if she becomes incapable of making decisions in the future?

13

- confidentiality. The gynaecologist may want to know about her progress and the results of investigations. Will Elaine refuse to let him know? Do the alternative therapists have a right to know as they are caring for Elaine? Are they qualified to interpret and act on the data?
- living wills and testamentary capacity. Who should bring out these options? When?
- resource allocation and financial problems. Is this an acceptable allocation of resources? What is the optimum interval between CA125 measurements? Who will decide? There are even more problems if the practice is fundholding.
- relationship with other partners. Will other partners agree to such a method of helping Elaine? What is to be done if they disagree? Is it appropriate to raise the issue in the practice meeting?

Thus, there are many potential problems when the GP is confronted with this situation. No matter what the final outcome is, the GP must make sure that all major problems are dealt with appropriately and sensitively.

Mr and Mrs Stirling have doubts about the diagnosis by a paediatrician of asthma in their 13-month-old son Peter. They refuse to use the inhalation treatment prescribed and have requested that they be referred to another paediatrician. Discuss your approach.

CONSTRUCT

- Review the circumstances
  - physical and psychosocial health of Peter
  - ideas, concerns and expectations of parents
  - reply from paediatrician
- Ensure good communication
- Promote better knowledge and correct attitudes to asthma
- Discuss diagnosis and treatment
- Discuss the request for second referral.

(Another possible construct is to list the alternatives in handling this situation and discuss the relative pros and cons of each.)

ANSWER

The condition of Peter should first be reassessed. Mr and Mrs Stirling are unlikely to accept any advice from the GP unless a detailed history is taken and a meticulous examination is performed.

The reply from the paediatrician should be reviewed. He should also be contacted by phone if possible. The reasons for making the diagnosis and whether and how the differential diagnoses have been ruled out should be investigated. How the diagnosis has been explained to the parents should also be known.

Effective communication starts with understanding. The ideas, concerns and expectations of Mr and Mrs Stirling should be understood. Reasons for not accepting a diagnosis of asthma are asked for. These can be poor knowledge, misconceptions and prejudice about asthma, communication errors with the paediatrician, a fear of labelling, a fear of the consequences, denial as one of the processes towards acceptance, or may be related to bad experiences such as death of a relative from asthma. A family history of asthma and atopic conditions should be asked for.

Adequate time, patience and an open attitude are essential when listening to the concerns of the parents and planning how to assist the family.

If necessary, books and journal articles should be reviewed by the GP before he sees the family so that the consultation can be more fruitful.

Mr and Mrs Stirling should be informed that very young children can have asthma, and that the presentation is usually of recurrent cough and wheeze with viral respiratory tract infections. A family history of asthma or other atopic conditions such as allergic rhinitis or atopic eczema is often *absent*.

They are told that a diagnosis of asthma at this age is based almost entirely on symptoms, and objective lung function tests cannot be validly and reliably performed.

Differential diagnoses at this age include cystic fibrosis, gastro-oesophageal reflux, inhaled foreign body, congenital lung abnormalities and congenital and acquired causes of immunodeficiency. If investigations have been performed to rule these out, the parents should be informed.

They should also be informed that although the response to inhaled bronchodilators is more variable at this age, this treatment should still be given. Preventive agents such as inhaled histamine-release inhibitors or inhaled steroids are used if attacks are frequent. The new four-step plan of management can be briefly introduced. It must be emphasised that inhaled steroids usually will not affect growth if closely supervised by a paediatrician, but poorly controlled asthma leading to repeated use of oral steroids will.

They should also be told that at the age that Peter is, metered dose inhalers with an extensor device and a face mask are a convenient and effective system of drug delivery. The inspiratory effort needed to bring the small drug particles to the small airways is slight and oropharyngeal deposition is minimised.

They should be asked whether they still have any concerns or queries about asthma and its management. Pamphlets about asthma in small children can be given.

Regarding the request for a second referral, rather than directly confronting them by agreeing to or refusing this, Mr and Mrs Stirling can be counselled on the pros and cons of a second referral. They can then make an informed decision. If they cannot decide immediately, they are encouraged to delay the decision, while still using the medications prescribed by the first paediatrician and carefully observing for the progress of the disease.

The family should be seen 1 or 2 weeks later to reassess Peter's condition and the compliance and technique of using the inhalation devices. They should be encouraged to attend the follow-up by the paediatrician.

A referral to a local asthma support group can also be considered at this stage.

The family should be advised that restrictive diets, unless supervised by a paediatrician and a dietitian, are unnecessary and undesirable.

After this incident, the GP may need to review his knowledge and skills of managing asthma in children under the age of 2 years, his interview technique and his communication with patients and specialist colleagues.

The first pregnancy of Mrs Brown, aged 32 years, ended in tubal pregnancy 4 months ago. She was anxious to know why this had happened and what she could do to prevent future ectopic pregnancies. What issues would you discuss with her?

CONSTRUCT

- Review the history
  - medical, surgical
  - OG
  - sexual history, use of contraception
  - history of STDs, cervicitis, PID
  - history of the tubal pregnancy, review hospital correspondences
- Assess present state of Mrs Brown
  - physical and psychological health
  - social support
- Discuss factors of ectopic pregnancy
  - at level suited to patient's level of education and understanding
  - emphasise modifiable/treatable factors
- Plan of management
  - discuss future family planning
  - possibly see couple together
  - further assessment and referral if indicated
  - good opportunity to discuss cervical smear.

ANSWER

The medical, surgical, obstetric, gynaecological, contraceptive and sexual history of Mrs Brown is first updated and recorded. History of STD, cervicitis and PID should be explicitly asked in an accepting and non-judgmental manner.

The hospital correspondence should be reviewed, including the histopathology report and preferably the surgical record. Details of the operation performed (i.e. whether it was salpingectomy, salpingotomy or a less common alternative) should be known as such affects future pregnancies.

The present physical and psychological health of Mrs Brown should be assessed. The recent relationship with her husband and the extent of social support should be known.

The impact of the tubal pregnancy on her family should be assessed. Was the pregnancy planned or unplanned? Will this incident affect her future family planning? Was there a history of infertility? Was this a long-awaited pregnancy? What is the attitude of her husband?

Mrs Brown's knowledge of ectopic pregnancy and related issues is then assessed. She should understand that an ectopic pregnancy is the implantation of a fertilised egg at any site other than the uterine cavity. In 95% of cases this will be the fallopian tubes. Other sites include cornual, fimbrial, ovary, cervical, primary abdominal and secondary abdominal sites.

Mrs Brown should be informed frankly that after one ectopic pregnancy, the risk of recurrence is between 10 and 20%. Thus, there is an 80–90% chance that she will not have an ectopic pregnancy in the future. (It is important to present both figures, 10–20% and 80–90%. Some people cannot perceive probabilities the other way round!)

She is informed that in most cases of ectopic pregnancy, the exact cause is unknown, although there can be some predisposing factors.

Advanced maternal age is one such factor. Thus, Mrs Brown should be counselled that if she is contemplating future pregnancy (-ies), it might be better not to delay too long.

History of PID is also a factor. Many patients (and doctors) are confused over the terminology of PID, salpingitis, endometritis, cervicitis, pelvic infections, etc. Mrs Brown should be told that PID is inflammation of the fallopian tube(s), possibly accompanied by inflammation of the endometrium or peritoneum, caused by infections ascending from the lower genital tract; it is unrelated to childbirth or surgical manipulations.

Most PIDs are silent (no symptom) or subclinical (minimal symptoms). Mrs Brown should therefore be informed that if she has had cervicitis, symptoms suggestive of cervicitis (purulent vaginal discharge, postcoital bleeding, deep dyspareunia), gonorrhoea or chlamydia genital infections in the past, she might have had PID and this may have been a factor in her ectopic pregnancy.

If Mrs Brown has history of PID or clinical examination suggests risk of PID, and this has not been properly investigated, she is better referred back to the gynaecologist for further investigations and management.

It should be explained to Mrs Brown that progestogen-only pills may also be a risk factor for ectopic pregnancy, as the tubal mobility is reduced. However, the use of an IUCD is not a risk factor. IUCDs protect against ectopic pregnancy, but are even more protective against intrauterine pregnancy. Thus, the absolute risk for ectopic pregnancy in a woman with an IUCD is reduced. However, if she does become pregnant with the IUCD in situ, there is an increased chance that the pregnancy will be an ectopic pregnancy.

Other factors that are related to ectopic pregnancy are anatomical abnormalities of the uterus (e.g. tubal diverticuli), history of tubal surgery, tubal adhesions due to past abdominal surgeries (e.g. appendectomy), history of ectopic pregnancy and assisted conceptions, particularly in vitro fertilisation.

Thus, in summary, the only modifiable factors in the case of Mrs Brown are advanced maternal age (which can be minimised), PID and progestogen-only pills.

It is best for the couple to be seen together for future family planning and counselling. This is also a good opportunity to discuss the role of cervical smear in the prevention of cervical malignancies. Education material on contraceptive methods and cervical smear can be given.

Mr Moss is 78 years old and lives in a nursing home; he has dizziness and recurrent falls. He is on the following medications:

- madopar '250' q.i.d. (total of levodopa 800 mg and benserazide 200 mg daily)
- digoxin 0.125 mg b.i.d.
- allopurinol 200 mg b.i.d.
- frusemide 20 mg b.i.d.
- thioridazine 50 mg t.d.s.
- amitriptyline 75 mg nocte
- nitrazepam 5 mg nocte.

1. What might be the indications for these medications?
2. What are the common adverse effects of these medications? Are any of these medications likely to contribute to his dizziness and recurrent falls?
3. How would you alter his medications?

(No construct is provided for this rather factual question.)

ANSWERS

1. Indications

Mr Moss is on a long list of medications. This is likely to result from the practice of adding a drug when a new problem arises, instead of carefully assessing the patient and taking him off unnecessary medications.

Madopar may have been given for symptoms of parkinsonism. Mr Moss may not be suffering from idiopathic Parkinson's disease, but secondary causes of parkinsonism. The commonest cause is drug-induced (see later). Madopar is not in fact indicated for drug-induced parkinsonism.

Digoxin may have been given for heart failure or supraventricular tachyarrhythmias such as atrial fibrillation.

Allopurinol may have been given for gouty arthritis and hyperuricaemia.

Frusemide may have been given for heart failure.

Amitriptyline is indicated for depression, chronic anxiety states, panic disorder, migraine, neuralgias such as post-herpetic neuralgia, IBS, psychosomatic disorders and insomnia. In this context, it is most likely to have been given as a hypnosedative.

Nitrazepam is likely to have been given for insomnia.

2. Common adverse effects

Madopar may cause GI effects, dyskinesia, postural hypotension and arrhythmias. Rarely, it causes acute brain syndrome, transient leucopenia and thrombocytopenia. As postural hypotension is likely to be a factor in the dizziness and recurrent falls of Mr Moss, madopar could be a contributing factor.

Digoxin has a long list of side effects, the commoner ones being GI effects, sweating, headache, facial pain, malaise, fatigue, drowsiness, depression, mental confusion, delirium, hallucinations and various arrhythmias. As the dose of 0.25 mg/day is quite high for an elderly person, digoxin is likely to be contributing to the dizziness.

Allopurinol can cause a maculopapular and pruritic skin rash. It is one of the causes of erythema multiforme and Stevens–Johnson syndrome. Other adverse

19

effects are GI effects, peripheral neuritis and alopecia. Unless there is objective evidence of peripheral neuritis, allopurinol is unlikely to be contributing to the dizziness and recurrent falls.

Frusemide can lead to GI effects, postural hypotension, headache, dizziness, blurred vision and hypokalaemia. The dose given is moderately high and no potassium supplement is given. Thus, it is likely to be a contributing factor of the dizziness and recurrent falls.

Thioridazine causes sedation, vertigo, postural hypotension and has anticholinergic effects. It can also cause parkinsonism and tardive dyskinesia, leading to the use of madopar. It is likely to be one of the factors causing dizziness and falls.

Amitriptyline causes postural hypotension with reflex tachycardia, anticholinergic effects (dry mouth, constipation, urinary retention, precipitates angle-closure glaucoma), drowsiness, dizziness, sweating and extrapyrimidal effects. At a moderately high dose of 75 mg nocte it may be a factor of the dizziness and falls.

Nitrazepam can cause drowsiness, muscle weakness and fatigue. Prolonged use leads to physical and psychological dependence. It interacts with alcohol and other hypnosedative agents. It is likely to be a contributing factor of the dizziness and falls.

3. Alterations

To determine how the medication should be altered, one must understand the problems of Mr Moss first. As he is on a number of medications that can have extrapyramidal effects, the parkinsonism is likely not to be due to Parkinson's disease, but related to drug-induced effects. Multiple medications lead to confusion, fatigue and dizziness. These then cause recurrent falls.

The following measures may help Mr Moss:

- The madopar should be stopped.
- The dose of digoxin should be reduced to, say, 0.125 mg daily.
- The dose of frusemide should be reduced gradually and the heart failure should be re-assessed.
- Slow-releasing potassium tablets should be given.
- Thioridazine should be stopped or reduced.
- Amitriptyline should be reduced gradually.
- Nitrazepam should be reduced by half, then stopped.

Clear explanations should be given to Mr Moss and the staff of the nursing home as to the reasons for the change of the medications. Communication and compliance are vital factors in the success of management.

Should there be any resistance, the GP can buy time by reducing the dosages of only one or two drugs very slightly first, re-assessing the condition of Mr Moss, and then reducing other medications very slowly.

The staff, and especially the night-shift staff, should be reassured that the behaviour and sleeping pattern of Mr Moss are unlikely to be adversely affected by the reduction and stoppage of the medications.

Janet, aged 13 years, consulted you for low abdominal pain, mostly on the second day of her menstruation on every cycle. Describe your management.

CONSTRUCT

- History
  - the pain
  - impacts of the pain, her ideas, concerns and expectations
  - urinary and genital symptoms
  - GI symptoms
  - medical, surgical, sexual history
  - psychosocial history
- Examination
- Initial investigations
- Treatment for primary dysmenorrhoea
- Treatment for other causes.

ANSWER

Janet is most likely suffering from primary dysmenorrhoea, which is painful periods for which no organic or psychological cause can be found. Secondary dysmenorrhoea, for which a cause is identifiable, and other causes of low abdominal pain, have to be ruled out.

History

The following aspects are assessed in the history:

- history of the pain – intensity (in a visual analogue scale of 1 to 10), frequency, site of maximal pain, sites of radiation, periodicity, exacerbating and relieving factors, response to medications
- impact of the pain – whether it affects sleep, schoolwork, sports or hobbies, and whether it leads to emotional tension, unhappiness and interpersonal conflicts
- urinary symptoms, including frequency, urgency, nocturia, haematuria, incomplete voiding
- sexual history, history of sexual abuse – although such issues are very sensitive, explicit questions and an empathic attitude usually lead to clear and reliable answers
- genital symptoms, including vaginal discharge, pruritus vulvae, intermenstrual spotting, genital trauma, dyspareunia if sexually active, anorectal symptoms
- GI and IBS symptoms, including frequent defaecation, pain relieved on defaecation, mucus on stools, abdominal distention, feeling of incomplete defaecation
- psychosomatic and PMS symptoms, including tension, irritability, depression, abdominal 'bloatedness', breast distention and pain, swollen fingers, headache and migraine, nausea, abdominal pain
- psychosocial history, including problems in school, problems in family, interpersonal conflicts, recent dating
- her ideas, concerns and expectations – why does she call for help now instead of earlier or later? what are her concerns about the pain? do her parents worry about serious underlying diseases?

- family history of primary dysmenorrhoea, PMS and gynaecological malignancies
- her surgical, drug and immunisation histories should be updated if necessary.

Physical examination

The extent of the examination depends on the history. If no particular underlying cause is suspected, general and abdominal examination and an examination of the external genitalia in the presence of a female chaperone will suffice.

Investigations

If no underlying cause is suspected and she had no pallor, a routine urinalysis to rule out urinary tract infection is adequate for Janet.

Any underlying cause identified or suspected should be appropriately investigated and managed; IBS and PMS are particularly common.

Management

If Janet is found to have primary dysmenorrhoea only, a meticulous examination and reassurance are already powerful therapeutic weapons. Otherwise, an NSAID such as mefenamic acid with or without an antacid might be prescribed to be taken when required.

It might be helpful to explain to Janet that period pain is caused by the accumulation of a substance known as prostaglandin in the body. Medications like mefenamic acid inhibit prostaglandin synthesis. They can stop the further production of prostaglandin, but cannot hasten the destruction of already existing prostaglandins. Thus, it is better to take the tablets as soon as the pain starts, rather than when the pain becomes intolerable.

In most patients with primary dysmenorrhoea, the above management is sufficient. Otherwise, combined oral contraceptive pills can be given for several months to regulate the cycles. Surgical treatment is almost never warranted.

If there is a strong element of psychosomatic complaints or IBS or PMS, psychological support with a course of TCA might be helpful. However, tricyclics are generally less effective for adolescent patients.

Mr Holmes, aged 84 years, had severe right-sided chest pain for 2 days. Examination revealed vesicles over the right T5–6 dermatomes. He also had DM and insomnia and was on oral hypoglycaemic drugs and a benzodiazepine. How would his age and past health affect your management?

CONSTRUCT

- List the aims of management first
- Physical
  — confirming the diagnosis
  — ruling out underlying conditions
  — antiviral therapy
  — pain control
  — anti-inflammatory therapy
  — hydration
  — complications: secondary bacterial infection, post-herpetic neuralgia, other complications
- Psychological
- Social
  — social support, admission, housework, meals, financial.

ANSWER

The susceptibility to herpes zoster rises with advancing age and waning immunity, which for Mr Holmes is related to his age and DM. I outline how his age and past health affect my management below.

Confirming the diagnosis

The diagnosis of herpes zoster is usually clinical. Investigations to establish the diagnosis are necessary only in doubtful cases.

However, because of his age and the probable presence of other risk factors, concomitant myocardial infarction and pneumonia are also possible. A resting ECG and chest X-ray may be needed.

Ruling out underlying conditions

The control of his NIDDM should be reviewed. If he keeps a diary of blood glucose levels or urine dipstick results, this should be examined. The drug compliance should be assessed.

The glycosylated haemoglobin level and urine for microalbumin might also need to be measured.

His age does not diminish the need for good DM control. However, this should not be achieved at the expense of a much increased risk of hypoglycaemia. Some practitioners might adopt a more permissive attitude to the diet of very elderly patients with NIDDM. This should be preceded by detailed explanation and discussion with the patient, preferably in liaison with a dietitian.

Other disease might also lead to an impaired cellular immunity. Depending on the history and physical findings, complete blood picture, serum electrolytes, liver and renal function tests, chest X-ray and microurinalysis might be needed.

Antiviral therapy

Acyclovir 800 mg five times daily for 1 week is the standard antiviral treatment for herpes zoster. New agents might also be given, such as valacyclovir 1g three times daily for 1 week.

In an 84-year-old patient with a history of diabetes an impairment of renal function is more likely. Upon review of past records of his renal function test results, a lower acyclovir dose might be given, such as acyclovir 800 mg twice or three times daily or valacyclovir 1 g once or twice daily. In general, dose reduction might be considered if the serum creatinine is more than 8 mg/dl, or if creatinine clearance is less than 15 ml/min.

There is no evidence that the incidence of side effects is greater among elderly patients. Mr Holmes should, however, be warned that common side effects include skin rashes, nausea, vomiting, diarrhoea, abdominal pain, dizziness and confusion.

If the general condition of Mr Holmes is poor, admission and intravenous acyclovir might be needed.

Pain control

An NSAID such as diclofenac sodium helps to relieve the pain. The dose does not generally need to be decreased in elderly patients, although an antacid might be given concomitantly. If cimetidine is given with the NSAID, the inhibition of liver enzymes may increase the blood level of acyclovir. However, because of the wide therapeutic index of acyclovir, the dose does not usually need to be adjusted.

Narcotic analgesics are usually not needed.

Hydration

Adequate hydration is particularly important for Mr Holmes because of his age and the need for antiviral therapy.

Secondary bacterial infection

Because of his age and DM, Mr Holmes is particularly susceptible to secondary bacterial infection, by staphylococci and streptococci, of the skin and the underlying tissues.

If there is already evidence of bacterial infection ('impetiginisation') of the vesicles and nearby skin, a course of systemic antibiotics adequate to cover beta-lactamase producing strains, such as amoxycillin-clavulanate, might be given.

If there is no sign of bacterial infection, regular cleaning of the lesions with sterile saline is needed. If the DM control is far from ideal, or there has been a history of recurrent infections, a prophylactic course of systemic antibiotics might also be given.

Post-herpetic neuralgia

More than half of elderly victims with herpes zoster may have post-herpetic neuralgia. For most, TCAs such as amitriptyline as a single night-time dose bring about much improvement. As Mr Holmes has insomnia, the sedating property of amitriptyline is beneficial. This can also replace the benzodiazepine that he has been taking, which frequently leads to physical and psychological dependence.

Elderly patients might be prone to postural hypotension and dizziness induced by amitriptyline. Also, they are more likely to have a history of angle-closure glaucoma, arrhythmias, benign prostatic hypertrophy, urinary retention and incontinence, and constipation. These are either absolute or relative contraindications to the administration of amitriptyline because of its anticholinergic effects. In such cases, a quadricyclic antidepressant or a serotonin reuptake inhibitor may be given.

However, the reason that amitriptyline can control neuralgia is partly related to its sedating effect. Newer nonsedative agents might thus not be as effective.

Should the control be inadequate, carbamazepine 100 mg twice daily may be given. In elderly patients this may particularly provoke confusion, dizziness and agitation. Thus it is wise to step up the dosage very slowly, starting from 50 mg once daily.

If the pain is still annoying, other measures feasible for elderly patients include other anticonvulsants (e.g. valproate), phenothiazines, butyrophenones or transcutaneous electrical stimulation.

Other complications

Post-herpetic paralysis and segmental muscle wasting may occur. Other complications include generalised varicella, pneumonitis and encephalitis. Another attack may involve other dermatomes and organs (e.g. eye, genito-urinary system). If these complications occur, management is very difficult because of his age and impaired immunity.

Depression is also very common after an attack of zoster in elderly patients.

Psychosocial support

Psychosocial support is particularly important for elderly patients. If he is very ill, has complications or if social circumstances do not allow adequate care and support, hospitalisation does more good than harm. Otherwise, he might be cared for at home, with home visits by the GP and the PHCT. He will probably need assistance with his housework, meals, cleaning and washing. Any financial difficulties should be attended to. The assistance of a social worker may be needed.

CASE 8

Mr Bell, aged 55 years, had his blood pressure measured by you on four occasions. He had rested for at least 15 minutes before each measurement. Phase 5 was taken as the diastolic pressure every time. The following results were recorded:

Date of measurement	Blood pressure measured on right arm	Blood pressure measured on left arm
14 Jan	165/90	160/90
19 Jan	186/102	184/96
25 Jan	150/85	Not done
2 Feb	176/92	Not done

List the factors that may have led to the variability of the results.

CONSTRUCT

Factors in the patient

- Physical and physiological factors
  - smoking, alcohol, drugs, food, hunger, fever, pain
  - arrhythmias
  - posture
  - support and position of arm
- Psychological factors, white coat hypertension
- Social factors.

Factors in the observer

- Systemic error
- Terminal digit preference
- Observer prejudice.

Factors in the instruments

- Sphygmomanometer
- Cuff
- Bladder
- Calibration
- Mercury column
- Stethoscope.

ANSWER

The variability of the results is quite large: SBP ranges from 150 to 186 mmHg, whereas DBP ranges from 85 to 102 mmHg.

The factors that can contribute to this variability can be related to the patient, the observer or the instrument.

Factors in the patient

Physical factors

- Although Mr Bell has rested for at least 15 minutes before each measurement, other physical factors might also affect his BP. These include smoking, alcohol, drugs (medical and drugs of abuse), food, hunger, fever, pain, discomforts (e.g. GI upsets), respiration and bladder distension.
- Another often forgotten factor is arrhythmia. Mr Bell may be having atrial fibrillation and his BP will fluctuate from beat to beat.
- The posture of Mr Bell affects his BP. For most people, BP increases from the lying to the sitting or standing positions slightly. For patients with postural hypotension due to autonomic failure, this can be reversed.
- Whether the arm is supported or not during measurement matters as, if the arm is unsupported, exercise is being done to support the arm against gravity, and the BP might be slightly elevated.
- The position of the arm matters. If the arm is below heart level, SBP and DBP are overestimated. If the arm is above heart level, they are underestimated.

Psychological factors

- Other than 'white coat hypertension' related to fear and anxiety when BP is being taken by a medical practitioner, depression, worries, fatigue, insomnia and sleep deprivation all affect the BP.

Social factors

- Social factors interact with the psychological factors. The BP is higher when taken by a nurse in the surgery than when taken by Mr Bell himself at home. It is still higher when taken by the GP in the surgery. If this is the first occasion that Mr Bell has met the GP, and it is for a consultation related to the CVS, this BP measurement may be the highest.

Factors in the observer

Common causes of observer error are systemic error, terminal digit preference and observer prejudice.

- Systemic errors can be intraobserver and interobserver. As the same GP measured the BP for Mr Bell on each occasion, intraobserver errors are implicated in this case. These can be a failure to distinguish Korotkov phase 4 and 5, poor hearing, unequal eye levels with top of the mercury column, lack of concentration and confusion of visual and auditory clues.
- Terminal digit preference is likely to play a major part in this case, as measurements taken on 14 Jan and 25 Jan were rounded off to multiples of five, whereas those taken on 19 Jan and 2 Feb were rounded off to even numerals.
- If, say, Mr Bell entered the consultation room one day smelling stongly of cigarettes, the GP might tend to adjust the BP measured to meet his preconceived notion that smokers have a higher risk of cardiovascular diseases and therefore are likely to have higher BP. This is an example of observer prejudice.

Factors in the instruments

- It was not mentioned whether the same sphygmomanometer was used on the four occasions. Different instruments of course can give different results.

Case 8

- The size of the cuffs and bladders may lead to errors. Too small a bladder causes undercuffing, leading to an overestimation of the BP.
- If an aneroid sphygmomanometer was used, recalibration against a mercury column should be performed every 6 months, otherwise there may be significant systemic errors.
- Whether the bell or diaphragm was used does matter. Whereas the results obtained from using a bell are more reproducible, a diaphragm covers more area and is easier and more convenient.
- If a mercury column was used, the column may not be absolutely vertical on some occasions, leading to systemic errors.

Fifteen-month-old Andrea was brought to your surgery for an MMR vaccination. She was born at 34 weeks as a result of preterm labour. Her corrected growth parameters and developments were normal. She had atopic eczema and infrequent episodic asthma, and her mother insisted that her eczema got worse when she ate eggs. Her uncle had cerebral palsy and epilepsy.

1. Andrea's mother requested a skin test to 'rule out' an allergy to eggs before the vaccine. How would you respond?
2. What are the contraindications for MMR vaccination? Is there any factor in Andrea's history that will affect her immunisation schedule?

CONSTRUCT

Egg allergy

The general approach is to:

- understand the ideas, concerns and expectations of Andrea's mother
- explain current guidelines for MMR vaccination
- explain difference between 'egg allergy' and anaphylactic attack
- take special precautions before and after administering MMR
- advise on other adverse reactions of MMR vaccination
- advise on diet and atopies.

Contraindications for MMR vaccination

These factors should be considered individually.

- physical factors
  - preterm and prematurity
  - CNS diseases, family history of CNS diseases
  - asthma
  - atopic eczema
  - growth and development
- psychosocial factors
  - parental concern, autonomy, informed consent.

ANSWERS

Egg allergy

The ideas, concerns and expectations of Andrea's mother should be understood first. She might have read something in the lay press that gave her true or misleading information on the adverse reactions to and contraindications for the MMR vaccine. Worse still, she might have known another child who suffered adverse reactions to the vaccine.

It should be explained to her that 'egg allergy' as symbolised by a worsening of the atopic eczema when a child is put on eggs is quite different from anaphylactic response to egg protein. An anaphylactic reaction is signified by generalised urticaria, swelling of mouth and throat, shortness of breath, hypotension or shock.

It should be explained to her that most paediatricians now believe that MMR vaccination should be given to children even when they previously had an

29

anaphylactic reaction after ingestion of any food containing eggs, as the benefits are likely to outweigh the risks.

Andrea's mother is then reassured that Andrea will be closely observed in the surgery immediately after the vaccination, in the presence of a doctor. In the unlikely event that there is any immediate adverse reaction, appropriate treatment will be given.

The GP should make sure that unexpired ampoules of 1:1000 adrenaline, hydrocortisone and chlorpheniramine are available in the surgery. Clear instructions for the management of an anaphylactic attack should also be immediately available.

Other adverse reactions of the MMR vaccine should be informed beforehand. Common reactions include fever, parotid swelling, rash and joint pain 10–14 days after the vaccination.

The relationship of the 'egg allergy' and atopies should then be explored. Andrea's mother should be informed that most children with atopies do not improve on any diet manipulation, and a temporal relationship between the food ingestion and worsening of atopy does not necessarily imply a causal relationship.

If the temporal relationship is genuine and repeatedly discovered, and the parents are highly motivated to try, a diet exclusive of eggs can be tried for a definite period of time, best under the supervision of a dietitian. Re-introduction of the assumed allergen must be included as part of the trial.

Contraindications for MMR vaccination

No factor in Andrea's history actually affects the decision to give MMR vaccination, although a history of allergy to antibiotics (neomycin or kanamycin) should be asked for.

The contraindications to the MMR vaccine are:

- acute febrile illness (vaccination should be delayed)
- immunosuppressive disease or treatment (but HIV infection and AIDS are not contraindications)
- history of severe local or generalised reaction after a previous dose of MMR
- another live vaccine administered within 3 weeks (although two or more life vaccines can be administered concomitantly to different sites)
- immunoglobulin administered within 3 months before the vaccine, or to be administered within 3 weeks after the vaccine
- history of allergy to neomycin or kanamycin
- pregnancy (although MMR vaccine given to a pregnant woman is not an indication for termination of pregnancy).

Preterm and prematurity are not contraindications or reasons to delay giving vaccinations. No adjustment is needed at all.

An evolving CNS disease is a contraindication for pertussis vaccination only. Epilepsy or other CNS diseases of the child or family members are not contraindications for any vaccinations.

Asthma is not a contraindication. In fact it is an indication for the yearly influenza virus vaccine.

Atopic eczema is not a contraindication. If there is extensive eczema, it is better to administer the vaccines at areas of eczema-free skin.

Andrea has normal growth parameters and developments, and failure to thrive (organic or inorganic) and delayed or deranged developments are not contraindications to immunisations either, unless such are related to an immunocompromising state or an evolving CNS disease.

Parental concern and anxiety are important factors for Andrea. Such must be addressed appropriately, or she might not be brought for further vaccinations. Any hidden agendas must be explored. The principles in counselling Andrea's mother are autonomy, advocacy and informed consent. The advantages and disadvantages of vaccination should be presented to her mother and the need for vaccination should be stressed. She should then make an informed decision and such decision should be respected.

Lucy, aged 5 years, has frequent episodic asthma with nocturnal exacerbations and atopic eczema disturbing her sleep. List your aims of management.

CONSTRUCT

Physical aspects

- For the asthma
- For the atopic eczema.

Psychological aspects

- Knowledge
- Attitudes
  — of parents
  — of Lucy
- Anxiety, depression
- Psychological preparation for treatment and prevention.

Social aspects

- Social life
- Diet
- Exercise
- Schoolwork
- Financial difficulties.

ANSWER

For the asthma, the *physical* aspects of management aims include:

- minimal chronic symptoms of cough, difficulty in breathing and wheezing
- minimal nocturnal symptoms so as not to disturb sleep
- infrequent exacerbations
- minimal need for relief bronchodilators
- rapid and good control of acute exacerbations (rescue course of prednisolone can be given if indicated)
- good exercise tolerance (the same or nearly the same as other children of the same age)
- minimal adverse effects of medications
- regular use of peak-flow meter to monitor (if she can cooperate)
- normal growth parameters, achieving the predicted final adult height
- no chest deformities (pectus carinatum, Harrison's sulci).

For the atopic eczema, the *physical* aspects of management aims include:

- minimal chronic symptoms of itch and signs of inflammation
- minimal nocturnal itch so as not to disturb sleep (a sedating oral antihistamine may be needed)
- infrequent exacerbations (which might be related to staphylococcal or streptococcal infections)
- rapid control of acute exacerbations and infections
- rapid identification and treatment of complications (e.g. eczema herpeticum)

- minimal side effects of medications
- no evidence of chronic inflammation (e.g. pityriasis alba).

The *psychological* aspects of management aims for the asthma and atopic eczema include:

- good knowledge of the conditions by the parents
- no denial by the parents
- a positive attitude to management of both Lucy and her parents
- good compliance and good communication with the PHCT
- no depression or unwarranted worries about the conditions by the parents
- empowerment for the family, no unnecessary dependence on professionals
- no fear of transmitting the eczema to other children
- a psychological preparation for her mother to breastfeed any babies that she might have in the future.

The management aims *socially* are:

- a normal healthy social lifestyle for Lucy and her family
- no unnecessary diet restrictions (unless recommended by a paediatrician and supervised by a dietitian)
- no restriction in exercises, particularly swimming, normal participation in noncompetitive and competitive sports activities
- minimal need for hospitalisation, minimal disturbance to schoolwork
- little financial difficulty, no housing problem.

The following quote is from the routine cervical smear report of a Mrs Maskrey, aged 35 years, G_4P_2: '...absence of endometrial cells, many polymorphs, mixed organisms with moderate inflammatory reaction. Inadequate smear, please repeat...'

Describe your management.

CONSTRUCT

- History
- Physical examination
- Further investigations and treatment
  — diagnose the infection
  — treat the infection
  — repeat the cervical smear
  — other aspects, including counselling and education, future contraception and the need for referral
- Review cervical smear screening programme.

ANSWER

History

- Elicit Mrs Maskrey's ideas, concerns and expectations, whether she has any specific fears or hidden agendas (see her and her husband together if necessary)
- Review medical, surgical and obstetric history
- Attain sexual history, use of contraception, history of vaginitis, cervicitis, pelvic inflammation, STDs, history of STD of partner(s), previous treatments
- Past cervical smear results, including dates, adequacies, history of similar inflammation, evidence of candidiasis, trichomoniasis, HSV infection, HPV infection, atypical cells
- Present and past symptoms of lower genital tract infection (pruritus vulvae, irritation, cheesy or greenish discharge, superficial dyspareunia) and upper genital tract infection (purulent discharge, postcoital bleeding, intermenstrual bleeding, deep dyspareunia, low abdominal pain)
- Assess Mrs Maskrey's knowledge and attitudes on genital tract infections and cervical smear screening.

Physical examination

- External genitalia: vulvae, Bartholin's glands, genital warts, discharge
- Vagina: evidence of vulvovaginitis, genital warts, discharge, pH
- Cervix: evidence of cervicitis (red and swollen, contact bleeding, purulent discharge from cervical os, strawberry cervix in trichomoniasis), ectropion ('erosion')
- Upper genital tract: swelling and tenderness on bimanual examination
- Other examinations: general state, breast, abdomen if indicated.

Investigations and treatment

To diagnose the infection

- High vaginal swab for trichomonas/candida smear with or without culture (if indicated)

- Endocervical swab for Gram's smear with or without culture (if indicated, special swabs for *Neisseria gonorrhoeae* and *Chlamydia trachomatis*)
- Other investigations and serology if indicated.

To treat the infection
- Treat infection if diagnosed
- Otherwise, a trial course of antibiotics is acceptable to control the infection before repeating the smear.

Repeat the cervical smear
- May be repeated 3 months after a course of antibiotics
- Ensure that the transformation zone is reached and complete 360° sampling is achieved.

Counselling and education
- Full explanation on the need for further investigations and a second cervical smear and the results thereof
- Allay fears (obsessions of cervical cancer highly common after an abnormal cervical smear report)
- Counselling and education on genital tract infections, cervical smear screening, contraception and other issues as needed, education leaflets.

Referral
- Refer to colposcopy clinic if:
  — second smear still inadequate
  — mild atypia on two occasions
  — moderate or severe atypia on one occasion
  — evidence of cervical cancer on physical examination or smear examination
  — evidence of HPV infection, including genital warts
  — evidence of HPV infection of partner, including genital warts
- Refer to GUM clinic if STD diagnosed or highly suspected, or if there is contact history of STD.

Review cervical smear screening programme

- Audit on percentage of inadequate smears in the past, close audit loop
- Review practice policy to increase cervical smear uptake
- Review practice policy of referrals to colposcopy and GUM clinic.

Mr Knight, 79 years old, could not sleep, woke up in the early hours of the morning and had had a poor appetite since his wife had died 6 months ago. He was flat and unresponsive. Everything seemed an effort for him.

1. Describe how you would assess the risks of suicide and deliberate self-harm for Mr Knight.
2. Describe your approach in the pharmacological treatment of Mr Knight, assuming that no organic disease is diagnosed on examination and investigations.

CONSTRUCT

1. Risk of suicide and self-harm

- Understand Mr Knight's concerns and expectations
- Assess his depression
  - severity
  - presence of psychotic features
  - factors
  - affect on daily life
- Assess suicidal thoughts and plans
  - attitudes and skills
  - direct questioning
- Other risk factors for suicide and deliberate self-harm.

2. Pharmacological treatment

- Principles of giving pharmacological treatment for depression
- Choice of antidepressant
- Assessment before commencement of treatment
- Monitor and document progress
- Cessation of therapy.

ANSWER

1. Risk of suicide and self-harm

Mr Knight's concerns and expectations should be understood first. His readiness to seek help and be helped should be assessed.

The severity of his depression should be documented. He should be asked directly whether he feels unhappy; helplessness and hopelessness in the future should be assessed. His appetite, sleep pattern, weight change and interest in hobbies should also be assessed. A clear picture of how his mood is affecting his daily life should be established.

Other than the bereavement, other predisposing, precipitating and perpetuating factors for his depression should be actively identified. Psychotic features such as hallucinations, illusions and delusions should be excluded, although this is not always possible in a single interview.

To assess for suicidal thoughts, the attitude of the GP should be warm, empathic and encouraging. He must be confident that direct questioning in such areas does not increase the risk of suicide.

Questions should be introduced in a graded and tactful fashion. The verbal responses and nonverbal cues should be noted and the pace of questioning adjusted accordingly. The appropriate use of the technique of 'silence' is especially rewarding in this case.

One of the questions may be 'Have you felt so low that it seems almost too hard to carry on?'; this could then be followed by 'Have you ever harmed yourself?' If there is a history of parasuicide or deliberate self-harm, the future risk is much increased. A referral to a psychiatrist is necessary.

If there is no history of parasuicide or deliberate self-harm, the next question may be 'Have you thought of harming yourself?'. Subsequent questions might be how, and then when and where Mr Knight has thought he might do this.

If he has suicidal ideas, ask about the plan. If he has a plan, ask whether he has already taken action, such as getting a rope. Ask whether he has written, or plans to write, a suicide note.

Other risks of suicide and deliberate self-harm, such as living alone, poor social support, chronic physical illness, alcoholism and substance abuse, should then be assessed. In any case, if there is any perceivable risk of suicide or deliberate self-harm, refer. This assessment should be repeated in subsequent consultations if needed.

2. Pharmacological treatment

Pharmacological treatment for depression should be initiated only after organic diseases such as anaemia or hypothyroidism have been excluded. The ethical principles to consider before the start of any treatment are autonomy, informed consent and advocacy. The patient has the right to accept or reject pharmacological treatment, if he is indeed capable of making such a decision. He should be given reasonably detailed information on the pros and cons of the treatment and alternative modes of treatment, although the GP can still advocate particular types of treatment.

A vast choice of antidepressants exists, from TCAs (e.g. amitryptyline), QCAs (e.g. mianserin) and MAOIs (e.g. phenelzine), to RIMAs (e.g. moclobemide), SSRIs (e.g. fluoxetine), SNRIs (e.g. venlafaxine) and SARIs (e.g. nefazodone).

No difference in efficacy has been demonstrated between the older and newer antidepressants. The major considerations are cost, side effects, risks of overdose and drug interactions.

In general, the newer agents (RIMAs, SSRIs, SNRIs and SARIs) are less cardiotoxic than TCAs. They do not cause postural hypotension or significant sedation and have no anticholinergic effects. SSRIs and RIMAs may produce significant nausea or diarrhoea, whereas SNRIs may cause hypertension at higher doses. SSRIs may cause agitation, anxiety, akathisia and sexual dysfunction.

In general, the newer agents are safer in overdose than TCAs and MAOIs, and drug interactions are rarer. SSRIs, however, may interfere with the liver metabolism of other medications.

Most of the newer agents are much more expensive. A practice policy may rationalise their use for selected patients.

The assessment before commencement of therapy serves to exclude relative and contraindications to the medication. For TCAs these include arrhythmias, pronounced ischaemic heart disease, motor disorders, recent stroke, glaucoma, prostatism and constipation. A CVS examination, including lying and standing BPs, is thus mandatory, and ECG and ocular pressure should be measured if indicated.

Some practitioners may give a very low dose of antidepressant such as amitriptyline 5–10 mg nocte, which can assure a good night's sleep without the need of benzodiazepines. However, antidepressant effects are not demonstrable below a total daily dose of 75–100 mg.

Mr Knight should be warned that althouth the sedating effect at night is obvious in the first few days if a sedating TCA is used, the antidepressant effect is seen only after weeks of treatment. The whole course of treatment, with regular reviews, should be at least 6 months.

If the response is poor after adequate doses and adequate time, a higher than usual dose of medications, combination of medications or supplementary treatment such as lithium might be needed. He should then be referred to a psychiatrist. Secondary medical causes should be reconsidered.

Nonpharmacological treatments (psychotherapy, electroconvulsive therapy) should also be considered. Good social support and assistance from the PHCT are also important in Mr Knight's long-term rehabilitation.

Augustine is aged 3 years and 6 months; he was brought by his mother and grandmother to see you. They complained that Augustine 'never eats anything' at meal times. Augustine's growth parameters are entirely normal.

How would you respond?

CONSTRUCT

- Understand concerns and expectations
- Take further history
  - dietary history
  - developmental history
  - immunisations
  - family and social history
- 'Child as the presenting complaint'? Hidden agendas?
- Examinations, investigations and referrals if needed
- Education and counselling
  - reassurance
  - snacks
  - food forcing
  - family pathology versus child pathology
  - see family together
- Continuity of care.

ANSWER

The concerns and expectations of the mother and grandmother should be understood first. It must be known why they consult for this particular problem at this particular time.

The dietary history of Augustine should then be taken. Attention should be paid to the number of meals daily, any snacks and drinks between the meals, any food fads and whether Augustine is being force-fed or bribed to eat.

The developmental, immunisation, family and social histories should be updated. Attention should be given to recent family conflicts, interpersonal crises and financial constraints.

The consequences of his feeding problems are then assessed. Feeding problems can cause much friction and tension in the family. The carers might be frustrated, helpless and depressed. They may feel guilty that they are depriving the child of essential nutrients. A high index of suspicion is needed to detect any hidden agendas, although they may not reveal themselves in the first consultation.

A detailed examination can be a valuable therapeutic tool. Augustine's mother and grandmother are not likely to accept advice and reassurance unless the growth parameters have been rechecked and the child's chest, heart and abdomen have been carefully examined. This should not be overdone though in subsequent consultations.

If any abnormality is found, further investigations or referrals will be arranged. It is most likely that no abnormality will be revealed, and his mother and grandmother should be told this. It is most likely that a paediatric referral will not be necessary in this case. However, should they push for a referral, it is best not to confront them immediately. A plan to observe and delay the decision to make the referral can be the solution of choice.

Augustine should be given no snacks between meals at all. If he is thirsty, plain water or diluted fruit juice can be given. If he is hungry, he should be told to wait until the next meal. If he cannot wait, a quarter of an apple might be given.

At mealtime, Augustine should be given the same food as the rest of the family. Food fads should be discouraged and no extra food should be given if Augustine does not like the food presented. His likes and dislikes should be respected though, and he should not be forced to take anything he does not enjoy.

If he refuses to eat, no attempt should be made to force or bribe him. No special attention should be focused on him, and he should remain in his seat until everyone else has finished. His parents should be warned that when they put this policy into practice, Augustine may show a decrease of appetite initially.

His mother and grandmother should be informed that Augustine is healthy and thriving. Mealtime is a happy social occasion and should not be ruined by force-feeding. They are told that they are doing a marvellous job with Augustine, who is not deprived of any essential nutrient.

Food refused is an excellent example of 'child as the presenting symptom'. The pathology lies in the family. All family members are unhappy, except Augustine, who is amazed looking at his desperate parents. His mother and grandmother should be encouraged to focus on other areas rather than feeding.

A strict dietary history does not need to be kept except in the most desperate cases, as it only increases tension at mealtimes. Should the family fail to cooperate in not giving snacks and not force-feeding, a session to see the family together may help.

Continued care is essential. A follow-up appointment should be arranged weeks later to assess progress and to iron out any difficulties. Other behavioural problems that Augustine may have, such as sleeping problems or temper tantrums, should be actively looked for and managed.

Mark, a 45-year-old executive, presents with pain over the lateral epicondyle of the right elbow. Tennis elbow is suspected. Describe how you would examine him.

CONSTRUCT

- Inspection
- Palpation
- Movements
  - flexion
  - extension
  - supination
  - pronation
- Tests for tennis elbow
- Tests for golfer's elbow.

ANSWER

A detailed history should be taken before the examination. Both elbows should be examined for comparison. Adequate exposure is mandatory. The basic sequence of look-feel-move should be followed.

Inspection

The following should be looked for:
- joint swelling
- muscle wasting
- equal carrying angles on both sides
- signs of past injuries and operations.

Palpation

- Localised tenderness over lateral epicondyle suggests tennis elbow.
- Localised tenderness over medial epicondyle suggests golfer's elbow.
- Localised tenderness over the olecranon suggests fracture or infected olecranon bursitis.
- The epicondyles and the olecranon should form a straight line in elbow extension and an equilateral triangle on elbow flexion. These relationships are disturbed in dislocations.
- Increased skin temperature suggests acute inflammation, e.g. infected olecranon bursitis.
- Palpate for loose bodies, e.g. lymph nodes, tophi, rheumatoid nodules, myositis ossificans.

Movements

All four movements should be examined. Active movements should be examined first, then passive movements with the examiner's one hand moving the joint and the other hand resting on the joint line, feeling for crepitations.

Flexion
The fingers should be able to touch the ipsilateral shoulder tips. The normal range is 145°.

Extension
Full extension should fully straighten the arms and forearms. Some hyperextension is normal. The normal range is 0–15°.

Supination
The elbows are flexed at 90°. Pencils are held in both hands and full supination is assessed. The normal range is 80°.

Pronation
The elbows are flexed at 90°. Pencils are held in both hands and full pronation is assessed. The normal range is 75°.

Tests for tennis elbow

The common extensors *dorsiflex* the wrist and *supinate* the forearm. Thus, pain is elicited over the lateral epicondyle (common extensor origin) in tennis elbow if:

- the wrist is passively (by the examiner) *palmarflexed* and the forearm is passively *pronated*
- the wrist is actively (by Mark, against resistance from examiner) *dorsiflexed* and the forearm is passively *pronated*
- the wrist is passively *palmarflexed* and the forearm is actively *supinated*.

Of course, there will also be pain if the wrist is actively dorsiflexed and the forearm is actively pronated. However, it is difficult and confusing to ask Mark to perform two active tasks simultaneously.

Tests for golfer's elbow

Even though Mark only complains of pain over the lateral epicondyle, golfer's elbow should still be examined for. It is less common than tennis elbow but the two conditions may coexist.

The common flexors *palmarflex* the wrist and *pronate* the forearm. Thus, pain is produced over the medial epicondyle if:

- the wrist is passively *dorsiflexed* and the forearm is passively *supinated*
- the wrist is actively *palmarflexed* and the forearm is passively *supinated*
- the wrist is passively *dorsiflexed* and the forearm is actively *pronated*.

For the same reason as above, it is difficult to ask Mark actively to palmarflex the wrist and supinate the forearm simultaneously.

Mr Field, a 38-year-old businessman, complained of intense generalised rash for 3 weeks. His wife and two children did not experience any itch. Examination revealed burrows on the sides of Mr Field's fingers and penile papules. Describe your management.

CONSTRUCT

- Diagnosis
- Differential diagnoses
- Further history
- Further examination
- Confirmation of diagnosis
- Treatment
  — education and counselling, pitfalls of treatment
  — treat whole family
  — choice of scabicide
  — application of scabicide
  — treatment of pruritus
  — treatment failure.

ANSWER

Mr Field is most likely to be suffering from scabies. Burrows on the sides of the fingers are highly suggestive of the diagnosis, and penile papules are virtually pathognomonic of scabies.

Differential diagnoses include eczemas such as asteatotic eczema or allergic contact dermatitis, pediculosis pubis, pityriasis rosea or systemic causes of generalised pruritus, such as cholestatic jaundice. All these should be easily differentiated from scabies by history and examination.

The medical, drug, travel and sexual histories of Mr Field are taken. Emphasis is given to history of skin and sexually transmitted diseases and history of drug allergy. Whether Mr Field has visited, say, his elderly mother in institutional care should also be noted, as this may be the source of the infestation.

Apart from the burrows and penile papules, other signs of scabies should be looked for. Burrows may also be present on flexor aspects of wrists, elbows, umbilicus and genitalia. There may be generalised excoriation marks and signs of secondary bacterial infection.

It is best to attain a microscopic diagnosis, as this will convince Mr Field of the need for treatment of the whole family and can enhance the compliance to treatment. A burrow is first identified with the ink test: a drop of blue-black ink is placed on the skin and blotted away after 2 minutes.

If the GP has a binocular 10X microscope or a very good visual acuity, the mite might be isolated with a flattened solid needle at one of the ends of the burrow. Otherwise, skin scrapings can be attained around the burrow and sent to the laboratory for identification of mites, eggs or faeces.

However, failure to identify the mite does not affect management as the physical signs are so convincing in this case. In all circumstances, treatment for the whole family has to be insisted upon.

The ideas and concerns of Mr Field must be understood before treatment. One of his expectations would of course be to get rid of the itch. He should be warned that the itch will persist for several weeks after successful treatment, as the itch is due to a type IV (delayed) hypersensitivity response to the mite or products of the infestation.

Mr Field may have other hidden agendas, such as whether scabies can only be sexually transmitted. If so, he might be reluctant (or overenthusiastic in some cases) to involve his wife in the treatment. The lesson is that unless his concerns are revealed and understood, treatment is bound to fail.

It may be worthwhile to remind Mr Field of the pitfalls of treatment even *before* instructing him about the regimen. The pitfalls are:

- one or two family members (usually the more elderly members) refuse or do not fully comply with the treatment
- not all areas below the neckline are treated
- scabicide is washed away prematurely
- all family members are treated, but not concomitantly, leading to reinfestation
- scabicide is re-applied as itch persists, leading to irritant contact dermatitis, and a vicious circle of assumed reinfestation and re-application.

Either lindane (gamma-benzene hexachloride) or malathion can be used as scabicide, depending on the rotation policy to prevent resistance. With lindane, there might be CNS effects and a small risk of aplastic anaemia. As it is diverted to body fats to be degraded, it is contraindicated in anorexics, trained athletes, epileptics, children under 5 years old and pregnant women. The latter two groups may be given malathion. The newer pyrethroids can also be used.

Benzyl benzoate is never a good choice because of the high incidence of irritant contact dermatitis it causes. Crotamiton (eurax) is less effective, and as many as five applications are needed. Monosulfiram is less effective and reacts with alcohol.

A hot bath is not recommended before application, as systemic absorption is increased. The scabicide, appropriately diluted according to manufacturers' instructions, is applied to all body surfaces below the neck line. The axillae, umbilicus, inguinal region, natal cleft, finger webs, fingernails, toe webs, toenails and the plantar surfaces are not exempt. For babies, immunocompromised patients and HIV-positive individuals, the application should be extended above the neck.

The application must not be washed away and is left for 24 hours. After hand-washing, the scabicide is re-applied. A second application is recommended 3 days later, although this is not absolutely necessary with lindane. Written instructions on the application of scabicide should be given to the whole family.

Mr Field is warned that the itch will persist for weeks after successful treatment, and a sedating antihistamine can be prescribed to be taken at night.

During and after treatment, continuous support is given to Mr Field and his family to ensure good compliance and the success of treatment. Apparent treatment failure is usually due to irritant contact dermatitis. Documented genuine treatment failure is usually due to incompliance. The whole procedure should be repeated after counselling for the whole family. Further treatment failure is either the result of a wrong diagnosis or resistance. The family should then be referred to a dermatologist.

Mr Goldstein, a 43-year-old labourer, fell accidentally and sustained injuries to both knees with wounds contaminated with soil. He was seen by you 8 hours after the injury. Describe your management.

CONSTRUCT

- History
- Physical examination
- Treatment
  - cleaning and dressing of wound
  - need for referral
  - anti-tetanus measures
  - systemic antibiotics
- Other aspects
  - education on wound management and tetanus prophylaxis
    workplace safety
  - vaccines storage and availability.

ANSWER

History

- History of injury – exactly when, where, how and why the injury occurred (clear documentation for medicolegal reasons); injuries to other parts of body; whether the injury led to a fall or a fall led to the injury; whether there was any change of consciousness before and after the injury
- Workplace safety – e.g. whether he wore a helmet; whether he followed safety protocols
- About the wound – the way in which it became contaminated and what the initial management was
- Immunisation history – whether he has had passive and active tetanus immunisation and whether they were documented (might need to check the documents or contact former GP); whether there were adverse reactions after immunisation; details of other immunisations
- History of previous knee problems (affects management as well as for medicolegal reasons)
- Other opportunistic questions later – e.g. smoking, drinking.

Physical examination

- General – conscious level and alertness, temperature, pallor
- Wound – site, extent, contamination, involvement of surrounding structures (e.g. tendons, ligaments, menisci, nerves)
- Quick examination for other injuries – upper limbs, back, head and neck.

Treatment

- Cleaning of wound – may be cleaned with sterile water or saline, finished with alcohol or hydrogen peroxide (but 70% alcohol is highly irritant to open wounds), simple sterile dressings
- Need to refer to accident and emergency department if wound too deep or involves important structures

45

- Anti-tetanus measures
  - The wound is tetanus prone as first, the injury was sustained more than 6 hours ago, second, the wound was contaminated with soil, and third, cleaning by Mr Goldstein himself may not have been thorough.
  - If it is documented, or if Mr Goldstein is reliably certain, that the last of a three-dose course or reinforcing dose of tetanus immunisation was within the last 10 years, vaccine needs not be given.
  - If the last of a three-dose course of the reinforcing dose was more than 10 years ago, and it is documented that the three-dose course was completed, a booster dose of tetanus vaccine together with a dose of human tetanus immunoglobulin should be given.
  - If he has not received any tetanus immunisation, or if his immunisation status is uncertain, a full three-dose course of tetanus vaccine should be given. Tetanus immunoglobulin should be administered concomitantly with the first dose of vaccine, at a different site.
  - The dose of tetanus vaccine is 0.5 ml, given intramuscularly or deep subcutaneously.
  - If there is no contraindication, diphtheria vaccine may be administered together with the tetanus. However, there is a possibility that Mr Goldstein is already immune to diphtheria. Thus the low-dose diphtheria vaccine must be used. Mr Goldstein should therefore receive either a tetanus vaccination or a tetanus and low-dose diphtheria vaccination.
  - A clearly typed or written immunisation card should be given, and a practice policy to call him back for further injections should be present.
- Systemic antibiotics – as the wound was contaminated and Mr Goldstein was seen 8 hours after the injury, a prophylactic course of antibiotics is probably indicated.

Other aspects

- Education – wound management, occupational safety, tetanus immunisation, educational leaflets
- Workplace safety – audit of recent occupational accidents, liaison with workplace occupational safety officer, liaison with district occupational physician, talks on occupational health
- Vaccines – availability in surgery, protocols on various active and passive immunisations, storage, audit of uptake, documentation of vaccination (practice-kept and patient-kept), practice policy to trace defaulters.

Mrs Hodge, aged 43 years, has been seeing several GPs and specialists for recurrent vaginal candidiasis. Describe your approach for her management.

CONSTRUCT

- History
  - including sexual and psychosocial history
  - expectations, hidden agendas
- Physical examination
- Initial investigations
- Treatment
  - conventional treatments
  - newer treatment methods
  - treatment for related conditions
  - treatment for partner (?)
  - holistic approach – education and counselling, roles of stress and immunity, empowerment, self-help measures.

ANSWER

History

- Vaginitis/vulvovaginitis – symptoms (colour, consistency and odour of discharge, pruritus, irritation), frequency, relationship with menstrual cycle and psychosocial stress, effects of symptoms (e.g. on work and sexual activity), past investigations and treatments
- Gynaecological history – including symptoms suggestive of cervicitis and PID, use of contraception (although use of COC pills is now believed not to increase the risk of candidiasis)
- Medical and surgical history, drug history
- Psychosocial history – family, work, hobbies, sex, smoking, alcohol, family history of DM
- Ideas and expectations of Mrs Hodge – hidden worries? misconceptions? fear of STDs?

Physical examination

- General – opportunistic screening (e.g. BP, breasts, varicose veins)
- Signs of vulvitis (erythema, excoriation marks), vaginitis (erythema, discharge) and cervicitis (ectropion, contact bleeding, pus oozing from os, 'strawberry cervicitis')
- pH measurement and KOH test of vaginal secretion for bacterial vaginosis
- Bimanual examination of uterus.

Investigations

- High vaginal swab for smear examination (polymorphs, yeast and pseudomycelia in candidiasis, clue cells, absence of polymorphs, small pleomorphic bacilli and cocci and decreased number of lactobacilli in bacterial vaginosis, wet mount for trichomoniasis) and T/M culture
- Endocervical swab for Gram's smear and culture
- A random or fasting blood glucose level to exclude DM is justified in this case.

47

Treatment

- Role of conventional treatment (imidazole creams and suppositories) explained to Mrs Hodge: they control the load of candida in the lower genital tract, but do not eradicate candida completely.
- Role of oral nystatin explained: it was originally thought that decreasing the 'bowel load' of candida might help, but this has been refuted by recent studies.
- Role of newer systemic agents (e.g. itraconazole, fluconazole) explained: they might eradicate the candida for a short time. However, recolonisation might be almost immediate.
- Role of treatment for partner explained: men do get candida balanitis. However, this is not likely to be sexually transmitted. Treatment for an asymptomatic partner is no longer recommended.
- Mrs Hodge should be informed that recurrent candida vaginitis is not likely to be associated with reinfection from other sites, is not sexually transmitted and is not related to the COC pill. Oral antibiotics might enhance an already existing infection, but would not increase the overall incidence. Altered host resistance is the key factor.
- Such altered resistance is related to impaired cell-mediated response, allergy and stress.
- Thus causes of impaired cell-mediated immunity, especially DM, should be ruled out.
- Allergy leads to activation of the immune system (mast cells and eosinophils), producing chemicals (IgE, histamine and prostaglandin E_2) leading to inflammation. Thus, Mrs Hodge is told to minimise use of spermicides, soaps and unfamiliar brands of tampons.
- Stress activates an endocrine gland (the anterior pituitary) to produce chemicals (elevated central beta-endorphin levels activate macrophages to produce further prostaglandin E_2), which again leads to inflammation.
- Mrs Hodge should realise the relationship between her life stressors and her vaginitis. Some patients experience a spontaneous improvement if they understand that the vaginitis is related to stress and is not a pure exogenous microbiological invasion.
- Otherwise, a period of counselling or referral to a clinical psychologist might help. If symptoms of depression are noted, a course of antidepressants may be indicated.
- Any concomitant psychosexual problems should be actively identified and managed. The couple may need to be seen together.

Thirteen-year-old Jane presented with breast asymmetry. The breasts were normal on examination, but a right thoracolumbar scoliosis (convex to the right side) was noted.

1. Describe how you would examine Jane and your expected findings, assuming that Jane had idiopathic scoliosis of moderate severity.
   Jane was referred to the orthopaedic department. Bracing was given but there was a plan for surgery.
2. Jane's parents were eager to do everything possible for Jane. What advice would you give them?
3. List the major factors limiting the development of screening programmes for child and adolescent scoliosis.

CONSTRUCT

1. Examination

- Inspection
  - arms, shoulders, scapulas, ribs, spine, hips
    upper back first, then lower back
  - inspection from all four sides
- Palpation
  - including the forward-bending test
- Movements
- Other examinations.

2. Advice

Advice should be given on the following aspects:
- roles of poor postures, exercise and heavy-weight carrying
- roles of bracing and surgery
- roles of other therapies
- prognosis and outcome.

3. Factors limiting the development of appropriate screening programmes

List Wilson and Jungner's criteria and apply to child and adolescent idiopathic scoliosis.

ANSWERS

1. Examination

Jane should be examined almost totally naked in the presence of a female chaperone when the GP is male. The steps of the examination should be explained. It would be ideal if explicit consent were sought for, although her turning up for advice implies consent for nonintrusive examinations.

Inspection
The arms, shoulders, scapulas, ribs, spine and hips are inspected systematically.
Viewed from behind, the right shoulder may appear more elevated than the left. The ribs on the right side are also elevated. The right scapula is more laterally placed than the left and is displaying a sharper medial margin than the left. The

49

gap between the right dependent arm and the trunk is less than that on the left side. The right arm may appear shorter than the left as the right shoulder is elevated.

This concludes the inspection of the upper back. It must be stressed that for idiopathic adolescent scoliosis, most of the signs are present but not apparent because of decompensation of other joints and postural adaptation. For an obese girl with a moderately severe curve and a compensatory curve, all signs can be missed if the examiner is not observant.

On inspection of the lower back, the left hip may be prominent. The flank creases may be more marked on the left side.

Jane should then be inspected from the right side. The left side of the anterior thoracic cage may be more prominent than the right.

She is then inspected from the front. Asymmetric skin creases and breast asymmetry can be seen.

Palpation
The forward-bending test consists of inspection and palpation. This is the key physical test in the examination of scoliosis of any type.

Jane, standing with both feet parallel and together, is asked to bend forward as far as possible. Her hands should be outstretched with palms touching each other, and should be pointing at the big toes.

The thoracic hump should be very obvious. The thoracic and lumbar scoliosis curves should be inspected and palpated. The inspection should be from both the back and the front of Jane. The erector spinae muscle on the right side is also more prominent and can be inspected and palpated.

Movements
The examination is incomplete without documentation of the range of movements (flexion, extension, lateral flexion and rotation) of the spine and the lung expansion on full inspiration. Percussion does not demonstrate any sign in idiopathic scoliosis.

Other examinations
A quick examination of the cardiovascular and the respiratory system, including measuring the chest expansion, is necessary. Her height and weight are measured and BMI calculated to assess for obesity (BMI > 25 kg/m^2, although strictly speaking, standard deviation charts should be used for adolescents). Her mental state is examined to assess for depression and effects of distorted body image.

2. Advice

Jane and her parents should be advised that:

- The curvature is *not* related to poor postures, excessive exercise, lack of exercise, vitamin deficiencies, calcium deficiency or carrying heavy school bags.
- Bracing might stop the progression of the curvature, but it *cannot* reverse the existing curvature.
- Physiotherapy, massage, chiropractic and osteopathic therapies have *not* been shown to have any beneficial effect.
- Electrical stimulation is uncomfortable, nonbeneficial and unnecessary.
- *No* restriction should be placed on her activities, except when she is wearing a brace, which may injure *others* in some contact sports activities.
- Close follow-up in the orthopaedic department is very important. If the curvature is allowed to progress, the cosmetic outcome, the final adult height, the cardiovascular system and the respiratory system can all be adversely affected.

- For most teenagers with idiopathic scoliosis, surgery is unnecessary and the outcomes of modern supervision and treatment are excellent.

3. Factors limiting the development of appropriate screening programmes

Whenever a screening programme is to be evaluated, it is useful to run through the criteria of Wilson and Jungner:

Wilson and Jungner's criteria (abbreviated) scoliosis	Limitations for screening programme for child and adolescent idiopathic
The condition should be important. For severe cases, scoliosis is important.	However, most cases to be detected in a screening programme are mild and the concern is mainly cosmetic.
The natural history should be understood.	More research is to be done.
There should be a latent or early symptomatic phase.	—
There should be a suitable test or examination.	—
The test should be relatively simple and acceptable to the population.	—
There should be facilities for diagnosis and treatment.	Most cases discovered are mild and no active treatment is indicated. Passive observation does not affect the outcome for most cases.
The treatment should be acceptable to the population.	—
There should be an agreed policy on whom to treat as patients.	More research to be done.
The cost of case finding, diagnosis and treatment should be economically balanced in relation to medical care.	This is a major concern, particularly in regions with tight budgets.
The programme should be a continuous process, not a 'once and for all' project.	Can be a financial burden in the long run. On the other hand, it is very difficult to stop a programme once it is started.

Thus, the major limiting factor is the lack of funds. It is also not known whether screening should be offered to girls only, or to both sexes. The optimal age for screening is unknown. It is probably around 12–13 years. The possibility of a two-tier screening process with a school nurse performing the forward-bending test and confirmation by a school doctor before notifying the family and referrals is being investigated. Otherwise, over-diagnosis may lead to both wastage of resources and unnecessary anxiety. Positively screened children might undergo unnecessary treatment, including restriction of physical exercise, if their parents had not received a clear explanation.

CASE 19

Mandy, aged 7 years, was brought by her mother Karen to consult for 1-month history of bedwetting. Mandy had been dry at night since the age of 30 months. What information would you obtain from them?

CONSTRUCT

- Define the problem
  - the bedwetting
  - accompanying problems
  - other problems
- Effects of the problem
  - their concerns and expectations
  - effect on home life, sexual life of Karen and her partner
- Symptoms of secondary causes of bedwetting
  - UTI
  - physical and psychosocial trauma, including sexual abuse
  - other causes
- Other histories
  - past health and drug history
  - developmental history
  - psychosocial history.

ANSWER

Define the problem

- Onset, frequency, and periodicity of bedwetting? Ever occur in daytime? Any precipitating factor (emotional stress, illness)? Does it wake Mandy up? Estimated amount of urine (any polyuria)? How does the family handle the episodes? Any rewards for not bedwetting? Any punishments for bedwetting?
  * A note on terminology: Mandy is suffering from secondary or onset enuresis, which means that there has been a period of normal continence without bedwetting. Primary enuresis is bedwetting without a preceding period of normal continence. Secondary or onset enuresis does not imply that there is a secondary cause, although the chance of finding a secondary cause, including emotional causes, is higher than for primary enuresis. Likewise, the chance of finding a secondary cause for diurnal enuresis (wetting also during the day) is higher than for nocturnal enuresis (limited to during the night). It is estimated that 15% of 5-year-olds, 5% of 10-year-olds and 1% of 15-year-olds have occasional idiopathic enuresis.
- Any accompanying symptoms? Any symptoms of periodic syndrome (cyclical abdominal pain, headache, nausea and vomiting)? Any genital symptoms (e.g. pruritus, discharge, urinary frequency)? Any behavioural problems? Sleeping problems? Relationship problems?

Effects of the problem

- Concerns and expectations of Mandy, Karen and other family members? Worries about particular diseases? What do they expect from the GP and the PHCT?
- How does the problem affect their family life? Does it affect the sleep of the family? Is the sexual life of the couple affected? What self-help measures have they taken?

52

Symptoms of secondary causes of bedwetting

- UTI – any frequency, urgency, dysuria, episodes of fever, loin pain, suprapubic pain, haematuria? As the absence of all the above symptoms does not exclude UTI, investigations to exclude UTI are mandatory in this case.
- DM – usually subclinical before episode of ketoacidosis. Investigation to exclude such is indicated.
- Diabetes insipidus – polyuria, polydipsia, neurological symptoms of pituitary tumour, family history.
- Epilepsy.
- Neurological disease – any faecal incontinence, soiling, difficulty in getting up from sitting position?
- Psychosocial, emotional and relationship problem – e.g. sibling rivalry or bullying at school.
- Child abuse – physical, emotional, sexual, neglect, Munchausen's syndrome by proxy? Symptoms of vulvovaginitis or STDs? Sexual behaviour inappropriate for age?
- Rare causes – renal disease, substance abuse.

Other histories

- Past health – update medical, surgical and drug history
- Developmental history – enuresis has many characteristics of *specific developmental delay problems*; however, such is applicable mainly for primary idiopathic enuresis
- Psychosocial history – recent changes in family circumstances, financial hardship, marital problems, problems at school, recent loss of interest in hobbies, other attention-seeking behaviour?

Mrs Bell was 68 years old when she was rehabilitated for myocardial infarction. She had been a piano teacher, but could no longer play the piano as 'playing leads to chest discomfort and weakness'. She lost interest in life. At her request, multiple ECGs were performed and showed no ischaemic change even when she was experiencing the chest discomfort. Describe your management.

CONSTRUCT

- Understand her concerns
  - hidden worries, depression
  - her expectations for the GP and PHCT
  - psychosocial stress, social support
- Analyse with her the impairment, disability and handicap
  - increase self-awareness
- Approach to future consultations and ECGs
- Approach to piano playing
- Future roles of:
  - herself
  - family members and friends
  - GP
  - PHCT
  - hospital physician and rehabilitation unit
- Housekeeping for GP and PHCT.

ANSWER

Understand her concerns

- Assess her knowledge of her physical disease. Likely prognosis? Any hidden worries? Family history of ischaemic heart disease? Close relative or friend recently having similar disease? Any misconceptions?
- Why is she repeatedly asking for ECGs? Is she lacking confidence in her recovery? Does she expect any improvement or deterioration? Or is it just a ticket of entry to a deeper discussion with the GP?
- Assess for depression. Recent mood? Hope for recovery? Have confidence in herself? Sleep disturbance? Appetite and weight changes? Other work and hobbies affected? Is she still interested in playing the piano? (She may no longer have an interest, but be projecting this to others as not being able to play.)
- Expectations of the GP and PHCT. What help does she expect from them?
- Psychosocial stress. Who is she living with? Housing conditions? Who is managing the cooking and washing? Is her diet sufficient? Financial constraints?
- Social support. From family, relatives and friends. Is there someone she can talk to and confide in?

Analyse her illness, impairment, disability and handicap

- Analysis of these entities gives deeper insight to both Mrs Bell and the GP.
- Her illness is ischaemic heart disease, presenting as a myocardial infarction, which is now in rehabilitation.
- Her impairment is chest discomfort and weakness, particularly when trying to play the piano.

- Her disability is that she can (or she claims that she can) no longer play the piano.
- Her handicap is that she can no longer function as a piano teacher.
- Active involvement of Mrs Bell in the analysis increases her self-awareness.
- Emphasise that the relationship between these four entities is not mandatory or unidirectional.

Future consultations and ECGs

- Consultations are useful for Mrs Bell's rehabilitation and for the GP to get to know her better. However, too frequent consultations are sometimes fruitless, lead to dependence in Mrs Bell, are disheartening to the GP and waste resources.
- A therapeutic or rehabilitation contract can be negotiated with Mrs Bell: she should contact the GP anytime if her symptoms suddenly change; otherwise, the GP will see her, say, once a month.
- Repeated ECGs reinforce Mrs Bell's belief that she is a cardiac invalid, do not affect management in most circumstances, lead to false re-assurance in some circumstances and waste resources.
- Formal assessments, including ECGs, will be performed by the cardiologist, say, once every 3 or 6 months initially. The GP will review such ECGs with Mrs Bell. Otherwise, the GP will perform ECG again only if there is sudden change in the symptomatology.

Piano playing

- A plan of rehabilitation should be established with Mrs Bell, the family, the cardiologist, the PHCT and the GP.
- Mrs Bell should be encouraged to take gradual steps in starting to play the piano again. On the first day or two, she might sit by the piano and assume the posture of playing, without actually touching the keys.
- Should she feel confident, she might step on the pedals on the following day, again not touching the keys.
- A scale or two can then be played with one hand and, later still, with two hands.
- The playing time is then slowly and gradually increased. She may then resume the confidence to play, and possibly to teach, the piano again.

Future roles

- Role of Mrs Bell – report any change in symptomatology to the GP and PHCT, maintain a positive attitude to life, participate actively in the rehabilitation process, communicate openly with family, GP and health visitor.
- Role of family and friends – continuous support, but not foster any unnecessary dependence.
- Role of GP – monitor her physical and psychosocial health, develop good doctor–patient relationship, facilitate empowerment of Mrs Bell, maintain good communication with Mrs Bell, PHCT and hospital specialists.
- Role of PHCT – home visit by GP or health visitor if needed, social worker for financial and domestic problems.
- Role of hospital specialists – monitor deterioration in cardiac function, tertiary prevention for complications of ischaemic heart disease, maintain good communication with patient and GP.

Housekeeping for the PHCT and GP

- How do they feel caring for Mrs Bell?
- What have they learnt through caring for Mrs Bell?

Mr Wilson, aged 66 years, is carried by his wife and son to your surgery. He is having an acute asthmatic attack. Under what circumstances would you admit him to the hospital?

CONSTRUCT

- Physical indications
  — life-threatening asthma
  — acute severe asthma
  — other indications
- Psychological indications
- Social indications
- Other aspects.

ANSWER

Physical indications

Admission is indicated if Mr Wilson has life-threatening asthma, or if he has acute severe asthma not responsive to immediate treatment.

The following features are indicative of a life-threatening asthmatic attack:

- silent chest
- central cyanosis
- bradycardia or exhaustion
- peak flow rate less than 33% of that predicted or his previous best value.

Note that pulsus paradoxicus is no longer recognised as a reliable sign of life-threatening or acute severe asthma.

If he has life-threatening asthma, admission should be arranged immediately. Prednisolone 30–60 mg intramuscularly or hydrocortisone 200 mg intravenously should be given, and nebulised beta-agonist should be started. In the ambulance, oxygen-driven nebulisers should be used.

The following features are indicative of an acute severe asthmatic attack:

- inability to eat or inability to complete sentences
- pulse rate over 110 beats/min
- respiratory rate over 25 breaths/min
- peak flow rate less than 50% of that predicted or his best value.

If more than one of the above features is present, admission should be considered. Systemic steroids and nebulised beta-agonists should be immediately given. If the symptoms, respiratory rate, pulse rate and peak flow rate are improved after the first treatment with nebulised beta-agonists, prednisolone should be continued and the peak flow rate should be continuously monitored. Mr Wilson should be seen in the surgery again within 24 hours, or a home visit can be arranged.

If, however, improvement is little or slow, Mr Wilson should be admitted to the hospital.

Admission should also be considered if the diagnosis of asthma is in doubt, if there are other concomitant severe medical conditions (e.g. congestive heart failure), if there are complications of asthma (e.g. pneumothorax), or if there has been recent hospital admission with previous severe attacks.

Psychological indications

If Mr Wilson or his carers are in a state of panic, very distressed and anxious, and have no confidence in monitoring and controlling the attack at home, the threshold for admission is considerably lowered.

Social indications

Admission should also be considered if the attack is in the afternoon or evening, and there is difficulty in monitoring his condition later because of geographical reasons. If the social circumstances are such that the GP and other members of the PHCT have genuine doubts about the ability of Mr Wilson and his carers to monitor and control the attack, admission might also be justified.

Other aspects

Should the practice possess a protocol for the indications in admitting a patient with asthma, such should be consulted. Guidelines of the BTS are also helpful and should be available whenever they are needed.

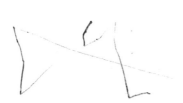

Mr Lee, aged 64 years, would like to discuss his life after retirement. He is a heavy smoker and has COPD; he is now on regular inhalation treatment. His wife is suffering from early parkinsonism. What issues would you discuss with him?

CONSTRUCT

- Understand his concerns and expectations
- Physical health
  — chest
  — smoking
  — CVS
  — musculoskeletal system
  — bladder and bowel
  — special senses
  — other aspects
- Psychological health
  — preparation for retirement
  — depression and related issues
- Social health
  — his wife
  — social activities and support
  — finance
- Other issues
  — health attitude, driving, use of health services.

ANSWER

His concerns and expectations

- What does he expect from this consultation? Any hidden worries?

Physical health

Chest

- How good is the control of his COPD? Does he have frequent chest infections? What is his exercise tolerance? Is he compliant with the medications? What inhalers is he now on? Has steroid responsiveness been established before the use of steroid inhalers? How good is his technique of using the inhalers? Does he have an extensor device?

Smoking

- How much does he smoke? Does he want to give up? Has he tried to give up? Is he aware of the hazards of smoking? Does he have the social support to give up?

CVS

- Apart from his age, sex and smoker status, does he have other risk factors for CVS and cerebrovascular diseases, such as hypertension, DM, obesity,

59

hypercholesterolaemia, a tense personality and a personal or family history of CVS diseases?

Musculoskeletal system

- Any joint problems? Obesity? How often does he need systemic steroids for his COPD (thus predisposing to osteoporosis)? Any mobility problems?

Bowel and bladder

- Does he suffer from prostatism, constipation, or incontinence of any kind?

Special senses

- Does he have good eyesight and hearing? Will either of these affect his fitness to drive?

Other aspects

- Diet, exercise, sex, other diseases.

Psychological health

- Is he psychologically prepared for retirement? Does he have any anxiety or worries about his retirement and future life?
- How does he view ageing and retirement? Does he have a positive attitude?
- Is he depressed? What is his personality before retirement? Is it likely to change after retirement?
- What interests and hobbies does he have? Does he have a good appetite? Does he sleep well?

Social health

- Who else are the couple living with? Where are their children and grandchildren? Will they be able to help in crises?
- Does he have to care for his wife all by himself? How is her physical and psychosocial health? Who is managing the cleaning and cooking at home? Is the help of a health visitor or a social worker needed?
- What are his plans for social activities after retirement? Does he have good social support? Does he belong to a church group or do voluntary work?
- Does he have any financial problems? Is he making good use of the existing resources?

Other issues

- In general, does he have a positive health attitude?
- What is his average alcohol intake? Is it less than 21 units per week? Other substance abuse?
- Does his physical health affect his fitness to drive?
- Are there local support groups for retired people in his area? What services do they offer?
- What is the future role of the GP and PHCT in the care of Mr and Mrs Lee?

Mr Thomson, 37 years old, has recurrent epigastric pain exacerbated by hunger. The pain occasionally wakes him up at night. He refused upper endoscopy because of the anticipated discomfort. Describe the range of options in the subsequent management of Mr Thomson and the relative pros and cons of each.

CONSTRUCT

- Aims of subsequent management
- Upper endoscopy plus other tests
  — pros
  — cons
- ^{13}C-urea breath test
  — pros
  — cons
- Serology for *Helicobacter pylori*
  — pros
  — cons
- Eradication therapy without diagnosis
  — pros
  — cons
- Combination of the above approaches
  — pros
  — cons
- Referrals and consultations
  — pros
  — cons.

ANSWER

The history is typical of a duodenal ulcer. Subsequent investigations should aim to

- confirm the diagnosis
- exclude other differential diagnoses and concomitant conditions, especially gastric ulcer and carcinoma of the stomach
- establish the status of *H. pylori* infection
- determine the sensitivity pattern of the strain isolated
- exclude complications of the ulcer, such as anaemia (unlikely in this case).

The conventional approach is upper endoscopy with biopsy for microscopy (stained with Geimsa), culture (microaerobic) and CLO test (urease test). The macroscopic and microscopic diagnoses can be made. Differential diagnoses are excluded. Moreover, *H. pylori* infection as diagnosed by culture is 100% specific and the sensitivity profile is available.

However, the procedure is uncomfortable. Spells of breathlessness may be experienced. Complications, though rare, might be worrying and prohibitive for the patient. Sedation with midazolam may be needed. The sensitivity for diagnosing *H. pylori* infection is not 100% (as a gold standard does not exist, the exact figure depends on which other tests culture is compared with).

Moreover, as Mr Thomson explicitly refused endoscopy, further advocacy by the GP might damage the doctor–patient relationship.

The sensitivity for *H. pylori* diagnosis is increased with the use of PCR. However, the specificity might not be 100%, as contamination might occur with biopsy forceps or the endoscope and thus, *H. pylori* infection would be overdiagnosed. Moreover, PCR for *H. pylori* is not widely available and is very expensive.

Culture may serve as a test of cure after eradication therapy. However, it is already difficult to persuade Mr Thomson to go through one endoscopy, and he would obviously object to another after treatment. PCR is not an option here as it is not established as a valid and reliable test of cure.

If Mr Thomson cannot be persuaded to have an endoscopy, a ^{13}C-urea breath test is an option. This test is fairly sensitive (around 95%) and specific (around 95%). It is simple, noninvasive and widely available to GPs. It is an acceptable test of cure after treatment.

However, apart from compromised sensitivity and specificity, the pathological diagnosis is not confirmed using the ^{13}C-urea breath test. Differential diagnoses cannot be excluded.

Serology for *H. pylori* is another option. Apart from venepuncture, it is noninvasive. It is generally less expensive than the breath test, and is much cheaper than endoscopy and biopsy for microscopy, culture and CLO test.

However, serology does not distinguish between active infection and past infection. Antibodies may exist in the form of IgG, IgA (less sensitive) and rarely IgM. In some patients, only IgA is detectable. Overall, the sensitivity may be as low as 36%. The pathological diagnosis is not established and differential diagnoses are not excluded. Serology cannot be used as a test of cure.

Another option is to give a course of eradication treatment (such as amoxycillin, clarithromycin and omeprazole for 1 week) without any investigation. As almost 90–95% of all duodenal ulcers are related to *H. pylori*, this is not a totally irrational approach. Needless to say, the differential diagnoses are not excluded as a test of cure is not feasible.

The above diagnostic options can also be combined into a feasible management plan with safety netting. One such plan is to perform a ^{13}C-urea breath test first, and treat if positive. After the treatment the breath test is repeated as a test of cure. If the initial breath test is negative, if there is no improvement in the symptoms, or if the repeat test is positive, Mr Thomson can be persuaded to have an endoscopy with or without ultrasonography of the upper abdomen.

This empirical approach is noninvasive and less expensive initially. The wish of Mr Thomson not to have an endoscopy is given respect. The test of cure serves as a safety net. However, this approach may give a false sense of security to both Mr Thomson and the GP, and the diagnosis of, say, carcinoma of the stomach, may be delayed.

Another empirical approach may be to perform a barium swallow and meal with or without a breath test and treat accordingly, followed by a repeat breath test as a test of cure. The pros and cons are similar to the first empirical approach.

A referral to or a consultation with a specialist can be arranged. The specialist has expertise in the area concerned, and the GP might learn from the referral. Care must be taken to prevent a 'collusion of anonymity' (in which no doctor is finally responsible for making an important decision) and an unnecessary 'perpetuation of the teacher–student relationship'. The pros and cons of a consultation versus a referral are too complicated to warrant a full discussion here.

One of your receptionists Barbara, aged 19 years, complains of suprapubic pain with vaginal spotting for 2 days. She is 8 weeks pregnant. What issues would you consider in your management?

CONSTRUCT

- The differential diagnoses
  - common
  - less common
- Immediate safety of Barbara
- The pregnancy and obstetric/gynaecological history
- The social history
- Courses of action and availability of resources
  - further management by GP himself
  - refer to hospital
  - specialist outreach clinic or hospital OPD
- Ethical and medicolegal issues
- Administrative issues.

ANSWER

The differential diagnoses

- The most likely diagnoses are threatened abortion, inevitable abortion, ectopic pregnancy, PID complicating pregnancy and UTI.
- Less common differential diagnoses are septic abortion, incomplete abortion, complete abortion, complete abortion of one embryo of a twin pregnancy, pelvic appendicitis, gastroenteritis and IBS.
- Uncommon and rare possibilities include torsion of an ovarian cyst, molar pregnancy, sexually or nonsexually transmitted enterocolitis or proctocolitis, inflammatory bowel diseases, herpes zoster, conversional disorders and drug reactions.

Immediate safety of Barbara

- Apart from the vital signs, including blood pressure and pulse, Barbara should be examined for pallor and surgical abdominal signs such as guarding and rebound tenderness. Admission to hospital should be arranged should her immediate safety be in any doubt.

The pregnancy and the obstetric/gynaecological history

Her full obstetric and gynaecological history should be reviewed, especially whether she has history of:

- previous or recurrent spontaneous abortions
- ectopic pregnancy
- pelvic and abdominal operations
- use of IUCD and other contraception
- PID.

63

The social history

- Is the pregnancy planned and wanted?
- Smoking? Alcohol? Use of other drugs?

Courses of action and availability of resources

- Barbara may be safely managed as an outpatient only if
  — the diagnosis is certain
  — surgical treatment is not likely to be required
  — the viability of the fetus can be ascertained
  — there is no evidence of septic abortion, sepsis or pelvic inflammation
  — admission is not likely to affect the outcome
  — the psychological status and social circumstances permit Barbara to be
    managed in an outpatient setting.
- To document the viability of the embryo, ultrasonography is most reliable. This
  might be available in the practice if one of the partners has a special interest in
  obstetric ultrasonography. It may be arranged in a day centre, as an urgent
  appointment in the specialist OPD, or at an outreach clinic visited by an
  obstetrician.
- Otherwise, Barbara is best admitted to the hospital for assessment and further
  management.

Ethical and medicolegal issues

Confidentiality
Strict confidentiality without compromising legitimate access to medical information
is difficult. A practice policy for the medical records of practice staff is helpful. A
code of confidentiality should be observed. Some courses run by organisations
such as AMSPAR (Association of Medical Secretaries, Practice Managers,
Administrators & Receptionists) cover the principles and practice of confidentiality
in the practice.

Consent
That Barbara consults the GP implies consent for history taking and general
examination. Should internal examination be needed, Barbara as a member of the
practice staff might feel embarrassed. She should be given every opportunity to
refuse examination. Explicit consent should be sought before the examination,
preferably in the presence of a witness.

Conflict of interest
* Sick leave might need to be granted. Conflict exists between the roles as
Barbara's GP and as her employer.

Administrative issues

- Should the embryo be viable, Barbara will need to take maternity leave in future
  months. The practice manager needs to prepare to cover her absence during that
  period.
- A practice policy may be needed for medical care for the practice staff.

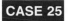

Nine-month-old Johnny had macular rash after 4 days of fever. You made the diagnosis of roseola infantum. However, Johnny's mother insisted that it was a drug reaction. Describe your approach.

CONSTRUCT

- Review history and physical findings
- Understand Johnny's mother's concerns and expectations
- Consider the differential diagnoses again
- Explanation and education
- Options and relative pros and cons
  — direct confrontation
  — authoritative confirmation
  — wait-and-see
  — seek second opinion.

ANSWER

Review history and physical findings

History and findings of present illness

- Onset and progression of fever? Onset, distribution and progression of rash? Other accompanying symptoms? Koplik spots in buccal mucosa? Occipital lymph nodes? Hepatosplenomegaly? Jaundice? Petechiae?

Drug history

- Any systemic drugs taken in the recent weeks? Any topical medications? Herbal remedies?

Past history

- Immunisation up to date? History of viral rash? Contact history with viral rash? Been staying in nursery? Recent epidemic of viral rash in the community? History of drug rash?

Understand Johnny's mother's concerns and expectations

- Why does she insist that this is a drug rash? Any hidden worries? Guilty feelings about having given Johnny any medications?
- What help does she expect from the GP?

Consider the differential diagnosis again

- Likely diagnosis is still roseola infantum
- Differential diagnoses include other viral rashes such as measles, rubella (but most with rash of first day of fever), infectious mononucleosis (rare at this age), parvovirus infection and, indeed, drug rash
- Depending on physical findings, rarer diagnoses such as immune thrombocytopenic purpura, viral infection associated thrombocytopenia, meningococcaemia, Henoch–Schönlein purpura, erythema multiforme, erythema marginatum and Kawasaki's disease might need to be considered.

65

Explanation and education

- Assess her knowledge on viral rash, drug rash and related issues.
- Explain to her, in a language that she can comprehend, the likely cause and progress of roseola infantum. Impress upon her that the diagnosis could not have been made on the first days on fever before the rash appears. Explain why other diagnoses are less likely.
- If appropriate, explain to her the role of serology for herpes-6 and herpes-7 viruses to confirm the diagnosis of roseola infantum (little use in uncomplicated cases, at present for academic interest only).

Options and relative pros and cons

- Direct confrontation: not likely to be able to convince Johnny's mother, damages the doctor–patient relationship and hinders further communication.
- Authoritative confirmation (e.g. showing her pictures and description of roseola infantum in a paediatric textbook, impressing upon her that the GP has seen many children with roseola infantum): might work if Johnny's mother is intellectually orientated, otherwise this can have opposite effect.
- Wait-and-see: impress upon her that time is a valuable diagnostic tool in clinical medicine. The rash, if due to roseola infantum, will fade in about 7 days. This approach can buy time for both the mother and the GP, but the mother might still not be convinced ultimately.
- Seek second opinion (e.g. another partner with special interest in paediatrics or a paediatrician): might convince Johnny's mother, but at the expense of time and energy of others. This might be the last option to adopt should all others fail.

Jane, aged 19 years, requests the 'morning-after' pill. From history taking, you suspect that she was raped the night before. Outline your management.

CONSTRUCT

- History
  - the assault
  - her past health
  - relevant medicolegal questions
- Physical examination and investigations
  - by whom
  - what to do
- Postcoital contraception
- Prevention and treatment of STDs
- Psychosocial support and follow-up.

ANSWER

History

As this is a potential medicolegal case, clear documentation is necessary. Jane should be offered privacy and encouragement. Empathy and patience in the interviewer are particularly important attributes for good history taking in this case.
   The following areas should be covered:

- her concerns and expectations from this consultation – is it just for 'morning-after' pills?
- past medical, surgical, obstetric, gynaecological and drug history, including STDs and substance abuse
- psychosocial history – smoking, alcohol, recent psychosocial stress, anxiety, depression
- previous sexual history, use of contraception, date of the most recent legitimate sexual contact and with whom
- date of last menstrual period, past menstrual history, type of sanitary protection used
- the most recent intercourse – date, time, place, with whom, any explicit or implicit consent on her part, any force, fear or fraud, any penetration, any ejaculation, any trauma, all other volunteered information
- any legitimate contact with suspect before
- her subsequent action e.g. washing, defaecation
- help sought up to now – family, friends, social worker, police?
- her expectations again – consent to inform the police or her parents? Counselling on the relative pros and cons.

Physical examination and investigations

By whom?

- By the police – Jane should be encouraged to report to the police. Late reporting leads to loss of trace evidence, healing or fading of injuries and can present problems for the laboratory. A forensic medical examiner will examine Jane and take forensic specimens.

- By the GUM clinic – a woman constable will direct Jane to a GUM clinic to assess for STDs. The GUM clinic might also offer postcoital contraception.
- By the GP – applicable only if Jane explicitly refuses to report to the police and to attend a GUM clinic. The GP is unlikely to possess all the skills and facilities needed.

What to do?

- To protect Jane against STDs the first set of investigations may include
  — endocervical swab for gonococcal smear and culture
  — rectal and pharyngeal swabs for gonococcal culture
  — endocervical swab with plastic handle for *Chlamydia trachomatis* culture
  — high vaginal swab for *Trichomonas vaginalis* wet mount and culture
  — serology for hepatitis B, syphilis and HIV
- The serological tests should be repeated 3 months later.

Postcoital contraception

The regimen

- The commonly used Yuzpe regimen is also known as CEP (combined oestrogen–progestogen). PC4 is one such proprietary preparation. It is ethinyl oestradiol 100 µg and levonorgestrel 0.5 mg given twice, 12 hours apart, and is effective for up to 72 hours after unprotected intercourse.
- The alternatives are postcoital IUCD, which is effective up to 5 days after the intercourse, and mifepristone (RU486). The latter is very effective, has fewer side effects than CEP, and is effective within 72 hours of intercourse.

Conditions for giving CEP
The conditions are:

- adequate contraception to be practised throughout the rest of the cycle
- adequate counselling (failure rate of 1–4%, possibility of ectopic pregnancy, small teratogenic risk, follow-up needed should there be low abdominal pain with heavy vaginal bleeding)
- no contraindications (history of thromboembolism, more than 72 hours after intercourse, multiple sexual exposures with the earliest more than 72 hours ago, history of ectopic pregnancy).

Prevention and treatment of STDs

The tests to be performed are listed above. If an IUCD is inserted, prophylactic antibiotics should be given. Even if no IUCD in inserted, antibiotics may be considered to cover gonorrhoea and chlamydia infection, particularly if Jane is unlikely to attend follow-up later.

Psychosocial support and follow-up

- The 'rape trauma syndrome' is a 'subjective state of terror and overwhelming fear of being killed'. There are four phases: an anticipatory or crisis phase of memory block, an impact phase of intense fear, an adjustment phase of anxiety, depression and denial, and a resolution phase.
- Some victims also suffer from post-traumatic stress disorder, with frequent flashbacks of the incident.

- Other psychological problems include low self-esteem, relationship problems, sexual difficulties and suicide.
- Counselling, pharmacological treatment or referral to a psychiatrist or psychologist should be considered where necessary.
- Jane's social support should be assessed as this affects the psychological outcome.

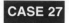

Mr Martin, aged 47 years, is planning a business trip to India. He has DM and is on oral hypoglycaemic drugs. What issues would you discuss with him?

CONSTRUCT

- Infections and infestations
  - food hygiene
  - immunisations
  - malaria
  - sex and STDs
- DM
- The flights
  - jet lag
  - air sickness
- Other issues
  - driving
  - the weather
  - availability of medical facilities.

ANSWER

Infections and infestations

Food hygiene

- Contaminated water and food can transmit enteroinvasive, enterotoxic and enteropathogenic strains of *Escherichia coli*, *Shingella*, *Salmonella*, *Campylobacter*, cholera, hepatitis A, hepatitis E, *Entamoeba histolytica* and *Giardia lambia*.
- Mr Martin should drink only boiled water or canned drinks. He should avoid unpasteurised milk, salads or unpeeled fruits or vegetables. He should be wary of seafood, particularly shellfish. He should only eat food that has been recently cooked.

Immunisations

- Recommendations on travel immunisations are changing constantly. Updated advice from either the London or Liverpool Schools of Tropical Medicine should be sought. Vaccination schedules are also published in *GP*, *Update* or *Doctor*.
- Tetanus and polio – given unless last of three-dose course or booster was given within the past 10 years.
- Typhoid – three types of vaccine exist: whole cell vaccine (two doses, 4–6 weeks apart), Vi polysaccharide vaccine (single dose) or oral Ty 21a vaccine (one capsule on alternate days for three doses).
- Hepatitis A – the single most important vaccine. Give a single dose of 1440 ELISA units. A booster at 6–12 months gives immunity for up to 10 years.
- Hepatitis B – given if his sexual behaviour is likely to put him at risk. Give 1.0 ml recombinant vaccine at 0, 1 and 6 months. A faster course of 0, 1, 2 and 12 months is also acceptable.
- Meningococcal – not usually needed. See updated advice.
- Pneumococcal – travelling is not an indication, but DM is. Two doses, 4–6 weeks apart, might be given.

- Influenza – travelling is not an indication, but DM is. Might give a single injection of 0.5ml.
- Rabies – not usually needed, unless for especially long journeys to remote parts where medical treatment is not immediately available.
- Yellow fever – not usually needed. See updated advice.

Malaria

- The choice of drug varies from place to place and from season to season. Seek updated advice. Usual drugs are chloroquine 300 mg per week or fansidar one tablet per week.
- Tablets should be started 1 week before departure and continued for 4–6 weeks after return.
- Other measures include mosquito nets, long-sleeved shirts and long trousers and insect repellents.

Sex and STDs

- His sexual history is reviewed and counselling given for possible sexual activity in India and the risks thereof.
- Condoms should be used. However, emphasise that these provide barrier sex and not safe sex.
- Mr Martin should be informed that most STDs, including HIV infection, can be asymptomatic in men and women. Should there be any need, he can attend the surgery after his trip for further examination.

DM

- Diabetic control is easily upset by travelling. Mr Martin should take regular urine or blood tests if necessary.
- The time changes involved in long distance air travel makes DM control difficult. If he is on sulphonylureas, hypoglycaemia is more worrying than hyperglycaemia.
- If possible, he should measure his blood glucose and adjust the dosage of the sulphonylurea. Otherwise, it is better to decrease the frequency of taking this medication on the days of his flights.
- An extra supply of tablets should be brought in case his return is unexpectedly delayed.

The flights

Jet lag

- Upset of the circadian rhythm not only leads to worsening of the diabetic control, but also fatigue, dizziness, nausea and impairment of mental performance.
- Mr Martin should maintain a good fluid intake. Smoking and alcohol should be minimised. Should he be suffering from significant jet lag, he should refrain from making any important decisions for 2–3 days.

Air sickness

- If he has history of air sickness, prophylactic medications such as dimenhydrinate or prochlorperazine might be taken half an hour before the flight, with regular doses during the flight should they be needed.
- If vomiting occurs, oral hypoglycaemic agents should not be stopped. The blood glucose level should be checked immediately.

71

Other issues

Driving

- If he needs to drive in India, inquire whether a medical certificate is required. DM patients on oral hypoglycaemic agents can drive unless their control worsens or they have frequent hypoglycaemic attacks, which is unlikely.

The weather

- UK dwellers might not be accustomed to the hot humid weather particularly in the summer months. Mr Martin should always keep himself well hydrated.

Availability of medical facilities

- It is best to check out the location, services and insurance coverage for medical facilities beforehand.

Nineteen-month-old Andrea has frequent temper tantrums and breath-holding attacks. Her mother Carol fears that she might die during an attack. How would you advise Carol?

CONSTRUCT

- History
  — characteristic features of a breath-holding attack
- Physical examination
- Diagnosis
- Referral, further investigations if needed
- Management
  — counselling and education
  — how to deal with a tantrum and a breath-holding attack
  — order, discipline and punishment
  — psychosocial problems in the family.

ANSWER

It must first be ascertained that the attacks are really breath-holding attacks and not epileptic seizures. Carol is asked to describe clearly what precipitates an attack and the time sequence of events. The state of Andrea just after the attack is also noted.

Breath-holding attacks are usually precipitated by pain, indignation or frustration. There might be a loud cry, and the toddler then suddenly holds her breath in end-expiration. She then becomes cyanosed. If there is still no breathing, the toddler loses her consciousness and then becomes rigid with an arched back and extended limbs.

Respiration then returns spontaneously and the toddler rapidly recovers. Characteristically, there is no prolonged drowsiness after the attack, as distinct from epileptic seizures.

Other relevant history such as medical, drug, immunisation and social history is then reviewed. Special attention is paid to recent family problems, interpersonal crises and financial constraints. Problems in the family commonly reflect themselves in symptoms of the child.

A detailed examination of Andrea is then performed. This not only excludes important underlying causes for the attacks (e.g. neurocutaneous diseases that lead to infantile spasm), but also serves as a powerful therapeutic tool for Carol. She will not be convinced that Andrea is physically normal if the examination is carried out in a rushed or careless manner.

A diagnosis of a breath-holding attack depends only on the account of the observers. Thus, if the diagnosis is in doubt, a referral to a paediatrician to rule out organic diseases is needed. Basic investigations will be performed for common metabolic causes of convulsions. An ECG will be performed as supraventricular tachycardia can lead to 'funny turns'. An electroencephalogram may also be performed.

On clarification of the diagnosis, Carol is asked to describe the general behaviour of Andrea at home and whether there exists simple systems of discipline comprehensible by Andrea. Throughout the consultation, the behaviour of Andrea is observed. Whether she is disruptive, hyperactive or has a short attention span is noted.

Carol is informed that temper tantrums are common in children of Andrea's age. In fact, the problem might increase in frequency and severity as Andrea approaches the 'terrible twos'. Breath-holding attacks in toddlers are also common, and are related to emotional upsets of the child, such as frustration or pain.

When Andrea sets off a temper tantrum, nothing can stop it. Any attention, scolding, praise or punishment at that moment is just like adding fuel to the fire. Thus, after making sure that Andrea is safe, she should be ignored. Her father and mother must not reveal to Andrea that they are annoyed or irritated by the temper tantrum.

After the tantrum, Andrea should be loved and cared for as if nothing has happened. She must not be given any rewards for stopping crying, or given any punishment for the tantrum. Any special response acts as a reinforcement for further attacks in the future.

As for the breath-holding attacks, Carol is reassured that Andrea's life is not in danger. The management is very much the same as for temper tantrums, and the parents and carers must not be manipulated by the child's attacks.

As long as Andrea can comprehend, a reasonable system of discipline should be established. Clear limits must be drawn on unfavourable behaviours. Rules should be few, simple and always followed by all adults in the family. This is, however, not easily attained, as the grandparents will usually break the rules and spoil the child.

When the limits of behaviour are exceeded, Andrea should be punished. The punishment should be immediate so that she can understand the cause-and-effect relationship. She must not be scolded or smacked. A peaceful period of 'time-out' is civilised and calming for both her and her parents. After the punishment, there should not be prolonged disapproval. She should be accepted and cuddled immediately, as if nothing has happened.

The basic rule is that discipline and punishment must be accompanied by love, or they fail.

Carol should also be requested to reflect upon the recent emotional and social problems in the family. At the end of the consultation, she is asked whether her expectations from the consultation are met.

Mr Wyman, aged 86 years, has a 6-month history of urinary incontinence. He has hypertension, osteoarthritis of the hips and knees and oedema caused by congestive heart failure. He is now on an NSAID, a diuretic and a benzodiazepine at night. How would you manage his incontinence?

CONSTRUCT

- Further evaluation
  - history and physical examination
  - investigations
  - use of bladder chart
- Distinguish between types of incontinence
- Define possible factors of the incontinence
  - physical
  - psychosocial
- Management approach
- Indications for referrals.

ANSWER

Further evaluation

- History: how frequently does he wet himself? Is it during the day or at night? Estimated amount? Does he try to reach the bathroom? Living conditions? Distance from bed to bathroom? Adequate lighting? Mobility problems because of his arthritis? Dizziness? Symptoms of postural hypotension? Symptoms of prostatism? Symptoms of UTI? Alcoholism? Use of other drugs?
- Physical examination: general condition? Nutritional status? Mental functions? Mobility? Neurology of lower limbs? Early signs of parkinsonism? Arthralgia and arthritis? Ankle oedema? Full bladder? Per rectal examination for anal tone and prostate size and consistency (though not predictive of obstruction)?
- Investigations: fasting glucose, microurinalysis, specific gravity, 24-hour urine volume, any other relevant investigations
- Use of bladder chart: very helpful in delineating the type and severity of incontinence. A sample chart is shown below:

Good Street Nursing Home Bladder Chart
Name of resident: Mr H Wyman
Name of nursing staff: Angela Moore
Date: 4 March 1999

Time	Damp, wet, soaked	Dry Volume voided
0200	Wet	450 ml
0730	Soaked	380 ml
1000	Wet	350 ml
1130	Damp	280 ml
1630	X	460 ml
2000	Soaked	230 ml
2230	Damp	140 ml

Distinguish between types of incontinence

- *Urinary incontinence* is the involuntary loss of urine that is sufficient to cause a social or hygienic problem.
- *Overflow incontinence* is the involuntary loss of urine as a result of an overdistended bladder (with or without an underlying neurological problem).
- *Reflex incontinence* is the involuntary loss of urine without sensation. A neurological cause is present leading to hyperreflexia.
- *Transient incontinence* is the involuntary loss of urine that is temporary and reversible once the precipitating factor has been identified and treated. This group has the best prognosis.

Define possible factors for the incontinence

Physical factors

- Excessive fluid intake – can be judged from the total daily urine output on the bladder chart
- Use of a diuretic – further increases the urine output
- Use of an NSAID – leading to fluid retention, exacerbating the oedema and necessitating the use of a diuretic
- Benzodiazepine at night – delaying his urge to void
- Osteoarthritis of hips and knees – mobility problem delaying his reaching the bathroom
- Other factors – e.g. UTI, alcoholism, parkinsonism, neurological causes.

Psychosocial factors

- Anxiety? Depression?
- Voiding habit – some people may wait for an intense urge to void, when it is already too late, before going to the bathroom
- Living conditions, lighting, slippery floor, physical barriers, lack of assistance.

Management approach

This varies according to the assessment results. The general principles are as follows:

- limit the fluid intake at night
- stop the diuretic if possible, consider using elastic stockings for the oedema
- stop the NSAID if possible, use paracetamol instead
- stop the benzodiazepine if possible
- change the voiding habit – remind Mr Wyman to attend the bathroom at regular 3-hour intervals, rather than waiting for an intense urge to void
- arrange easy access to the bathroom, arrange assistance if needed
- education and support to Mr Wyman and his carers.

Indications for referral

- Treatable physical cause identified – e.g. severe prostatism
- Unknown neurological cause – admit for investigations e.g. CT scan of brain
- Severe depression, suicidal tendency
- Condition deteriorating despite treatment
- Patient and carers can no longer cope
- Neglect or abuse suspected.

You think that you are depressed and have experienced a burnout. Who would you turn to for help? What are the pros and cons of turning to them for help?

CONSTRUCT

- Spouse, family, friends
- Partners
- PHCT
- GP
- Psychiatrist, psychologist.

ANSWER

In this case, the GP is the patient himself. His help-seeking behaviour may be quite different from other patients, and there can be problems such as capability to continue working as a GP and conflict of roles.

The GP can turn to his spouse and family for help. They can offer him emotional support. Good family and social support is important for recovering from a burnout.

However, unless the spouse is also a medical practitioner, she will not be in a position to make a diagnosis, assess the severity and comment on management. If the spouse is a medical practitioner, there can be role conflicts that can adversely affect the future help-seeking behaviour of the GP.

The GP can turn to his partners. The partner can make a diagnosis, assess the severity and manage the psychological problems. Having been working with the GP for some time, he might have personal knowledge of the joys and pains of the GP that no other practitioner possesses.

Moreover, as the psychological problems might affect the GP's capability to work, the partner can plan ahead for the future workload and time off.

However, the partner's assessment may not be totally impartial, as there is a conflict of interest with regard to workload and time off. Moreover, the roles will be confused, changing from the normal adult–adult interaction between partners to doctor–patient or parent–child interactions.

The GP may turn to members of the PHCT for help. They can give him support. They can re-arrange the workload, such as child health clinics and home visits, so that the GP can take a break in the short term.

However, if the PHCT is involved, the GP may be stigmatised as having a psychological problem. This can affect the working relationship between the GP and the PHCT members, who may also lose confidence in the working capability of the GP.

The GP should turn to his own GP, preferably not in the same practice, for help. If the GP believes in the values of continuity of care and a health doctor–patient relationship, he will believe that advice from his own GP is invaluable. The doctor–patient relationship is clear and there is no role conflict.

The GP of the GP can assess the GP objectively and impartially. He can offer counselling and psychological support. Drug and substance abuse is common in the medical profession. If pharmacological treatment is needed, he can supervise the GP to prevent abuse and dependence. He can initiate a referral to a psychiatrist if needed.

However, the GP of the GP may not have a special interest in psychological problems. It can be embarrassing if his expertise in dealing with these problems is far less than that of the consulting GP. Also, if the GP of the GP thinks that the consulting GP is not capable of offering care to his patients, he will find himself in a very difficult position.

How about consulting a psychiatrist directly? Obviously, the psychiatrist has the expertise to help the GP and can offer continuity of care provided the GP stays with the same psychiatrist in the long run. The doctor–patient relationship is clear, although there can be an element of perpetuation of the teacher–student relationship.

However, this strategy bypasses the primary care stratum. If the gatekeeper role of the GP is not respected by the GP himself, how can he expect his patients to respect the importance of primary care? Moreover, underlying organic causes for the depression, such as hypothyroidism, have not been excluded before the secondary care consultation.

The GP may also consult a clinical psychologist or a counsellor directly. The pros and cons are similar to those for consulting a psychiatrist directly, except that the danger of omitting organic diagnoses is even greater.

In conclusion, there are many people to whom the GP can turn for advice and help. If he believes in the importance of the GP in the health care system, he should consult his own GP who should offer the same continuous high quality primary care to him as to any other patient.

Mrs Desmond, aged 58 years, has requested that an ABPM be arranged for her for insurance purposes. She has borderline HT and has not been put on any antihypertensive agents. She has offered to settle all costs incurred. What factors affect your response?

CONSTRUCT

- Factors related to Mrs Desmond
  - past health, risk factors for CVS and cerebrovascular diseases
  - her BP record and measurements
  - her insurance
  - her concerns and expectations
  - the ABPM and the report
- Factors related to the practice
  - availability of equipment
  - benefits for other patients
  - financial resources of the practice
- Factors related to the GP
  - expertise on BP measurement and ABPM
  - protocol for BP measurement and treatment of HT
  - audit for BP measurement and treatment of HT.

ANSWER

Factors related to Mrs Desmond

- Review medical and drug history: other risk factors for CVS and cerebrovascular diseases (smoking, hypercholesterolaemia, DM, obesity, lack of exercise, tense personality, family history)? History of HRT?
- Review all past BP measurements: measured by whom and how often? What indication? Enough time to relax and rest? Obvious systemic error, terminal digit preference or observer prejudice? Was phase IV or phase V used? Why?
- The insurance: was she penalised for insurance coverage because of HT? Who took the BP on behalf of the insurance company? Under what circumstances? Were the measurements repeated?
- The ABPM: who suggested this to her? Is an ABPM likely to benefit her medically? What if the ABPM reveals unfavourable results? Will she still send the report to the insurance company? Will she pay if the results are unfavourable? Is the report urgently needed?
- Other concerns and expectations: any other ways to help her?

Factors related to the practice

- Most practices do not have the equipment for ABPM. The device might have to be purchased or leased, or Mrs Desmond be referred to other practices or a specialist.
- Will the purchase of such equipment be a good investment? Common indications for ABPM include borderline HT, isolated systolic HT in the elderly, suspected nocturnal HT, suspected symptomatic HT, and to differentiate 'white coat' HT from genuine HT. Are there many such patients on the practice list? Will ABPM affect the management of these patients?

79

- If money is taken from the budget to purchase ABPM equipment, less resources will be available in other areas. Is ABPM the best area of resource allocation? Is it cost effective?
- What is the approximate cost? Which devices have fulfilled the criteria of the British Hypertension Society? Are there maintenance costs?
- Will the expense be reimbursed? Will other partners agree? Should the issue be raised in the practice meeting?

Factors related to the GP

- What do I know about ABPM myself? Will other partners and I be able to interpret the resulting BP measurements? Where can I obtain further information?
- Will ABPM give a clearer answer to patients in the 'grey zone'? Or will it lead to even more confusion?
- Does the practice have a protocol for BP measurement and HT management? When was it drafted? Is it due for a review?
- How would ABPM be fitted into the HT protocol?
- Has an audit for BP measurement and HT treatment been performed? Was the audit loop closed?

Mrs Maclean presents with pruritic scaly lesions on the trunk that are unresponsive to local empirical treatments. A diagnostic punch biopsy is to be performed. Draft a consent form for the procedure.

CONSTRUCT

- Patient data
- Indication and type of minor surgery
- Simple description of procedure
- Risks
- Informed consent
- Signatures.

ANSWER

The Bonham Surgery Minor Surgery Consent Form

Patient name:

Sex:

Age:

Registration number:

Date of surgery:

I consent to the following surgery: (diagnostic punch biopsy for scaly skin lesions on the trunk)
The exact procedures have been explained to me as: (giving local anaesthesia, getting a cylindrical section of skin and related structures, and sewing it up)
I understand that the risks might include: (scarring, bleeding, infection, and an allergic reaction to the anaesthetic agent)
I have had an opportunity to ask all questions about the minor surgery, and I was informed of other modes of treatment and diagnosis.
Patient signature:
Witness signature:
GP signature:

Mrs Martin, aged 49 years, has been suffering from cervical spondylosis for years. What factors might affect the severity and frequency of her symptoms?

CONSTRUCT

- Physical factors
  - extent and severity of the disease
  - effects of other structures
  - other physical factors
- Psychological factors
- Social factors.

ANSWER

Physical factors

- Extent, severity and chronicity of the disease (however, the radiological changes are not directly proportional to the severity of symptoms)
- Effects on other structures
  - locally: central neck pain that may radiate to the occiput, occipital headache, pain exacerbated by neck movements, restriction of neck movements
  - nerve root: pain radiating to shoulders, arms and hands, muscle weakness, parasthesia (examination will reveal signs of lower motor neuron lesion)
  - spinal cord: unsteady gait (examination revealing signs of upper motor neuron lesion)
  - vertebral artery: drop attacks precipitated by neck extension
  - oesophagus: dysphagia (rare)
- Accompanying osteoporosis (no pain unless with fractures) and osteomalacia (associated with pain)
- Presence of other musculoskeletal diseases, e.g. rheumatoid arthritis
- Hormonal status, e.g. premature surgical menopause with no HRT
- Diet and exercise
- Medications, physiotherapy, message, other manipulative therapies (e.g. chiropractic, osteopathy).

Psychological factors

- Personal attitude and philosophy to chronic pain
- Pain threshold
- Secondary gains from the pain (e.g. sick leaves), attention-seeking behaviour
- Menopausal symptoms (e.g. empty nest syndrome)
- Anxiety, irritability, depression
- Quality of relaxation and sleep.

Social factors

- Social support (family, friends), relationship with family members
- Social activities, interests and hobbies
- A competent and compassionate GP
- Support from the PHCT
- Holistic pain clinic
- Local support group.

William, aged 10 years, has a height of 135 cm and a weight of 48.5 kg.

1. Given that the 95th percentile for the BMI of boys at 10 years of age is 23 kg/m², calculate and comment on the BMI of William.
2. What complications might William be prone to?
3. List your preventive strategies for childhood and adolescent obesity and its complications.

CONSTRUCT

1. BMI

● Calculate BMI
● Interpret BMI.

2. Complications

● Physical
 — CVS
 — respiratory
 — CNS
 — endocrine
 — hepatobiliary
 — musculoskeletal
● Psychological
● Social.

3. Preventive strategies

● Primary prevention
● Secondary prevention
● Tertiary prevention.

ANSWERS

1. BMI

BMI = Body weight in kg/(Height in m)² = 26.6 kg/m²

Children and adolescents with BMIs at the 95th percentile or more for their age and sex or whose BMIs are more than 30 kg/m² (unlike adults, for whom 25 kg/m² is the dividing line) can be said to be overweight. Thus, William is regarded as being overweight.

The same conclusion can be reached on the growth percentile charts, as William's height is near the 50th percentile whereas his weight is at the 97th percentile.

2. Complications

Physical complications

● CVS: hypertension, hypercholesterolaemia, hypertriglyceridaemia, LDL hyperlipoproteinaemia, VLDL hyperlipoproteinaemia, HDL hypolipoproteinaemia
● Respiratory: frequent respiratory tract infections, abnormal lung function tests, Pickwickian syndrome (hypoxaemia, central cyanosis, polycythaemia, congestive heart failure)

- CNS: pseudotumour cerebri (raised intracranial pressure, normal CSF biochemistry and cell counts, normal CNS anatomy)
- Endocrine system: DM
- Hepatobiliary: cholelithiasis
- Musculoskeletal: Blount's disease, Perthes' disease, slipped femoral epiphyses. However, most children and adolescents with obesity do not have any physical complication.

Psychological complications

- Depression, anxiety (e.g. because of apparently small external genitalia).
  Social complications
- Family conflicts (over the need for diet restrictions or not), teasing by schoolmates, isolation by peers.

3. Preventive strategies

Primary prevention

- Health education by GP and other members of PHCT, especially health visitors
- Posters and leaflets on prevention of child and adolescent obesity
- Encourage breastfeeding
- Central message of healthy eating
  — children should only eat when hungry
  — no snack between proper meals
  — scheduled time for proper meals
  — children have the option to eat or not
  — no force-feeding, no bribes
  — change of eating habit for the whole family, not just the child
  — five food groups (two helpings daily from meat group, one pint full-cream or semi-skimmed milk daily for children aged over 5 years, five different kinds of fruits and vegetables, cereals at meal times only, small quantities of fat).

Secondary prevention

- Opportunistic screening (weight and BMI) for apparently overweight children and adolescents
- Role of mass screening programmes uncertain
- Screening for high risk groups: family history of obesity, mentally retarded, several syndromes (Turner's, Prader–Willi, Lawrence–Moon–Biedl).

Tertiary prevention

- Early treatment of identified cases to prevent complications
- Diet control supervised by dietitian
- Regular exercise, for the whole family
- Early referral of resistant cases to a paediatrician with special interest in growth and obesity
- Early detection of complications, e.g. hyperlipidaemias, hypertension, slipped femoral epiphyses
- Early treatment and referral for complications.

Mrs Lewis, aged 44 years, is getting married for the second time next month. Her two children, aged 15 and 17 years, are healthy. She is not planning to have further children and consults you about her contraceptive needs. Describe your management.

CONSTRUCT

- History
- Physical examination
- Choice of contraceptive method
  — principles of contraceptive counselling
  — the criteria for a good contraceptive method
  — the various methods, including sterilisation.

ANSWER

History

- Her concerns and expectations, hidden worries
- Past medical, surgical, obstetric, menstrual and sexual history
- History of gynaecological diseases, pelvic infections and STDs
- History of use of contraception, reasons for the choice, acceptability, adverse reactions, history of failure, acceptability to partner, reason to change, compliance, her knowledge of and attitudes to other methods
- Drug history, drug allergy
- Psychosocial history, including use of tobacco and alcohol
- Family history, especially history of carcinoma of the breast and thromboembolism.

Physical examination

- Height, weight, BMI
- Varicose veins, CVS, BP
- Breast, abdomen
- Pelvic examination, cervical smear if due
- Microurinalysis with or without fasting glucose.

Choice of contraceptive method

- Principles of contraceptive counselling: autonomy, informed choice, advocacy. Mrs Lewis must be clear about the roles played by the GP: it is her own choice, not the GP's.
- Criteria of a good contraceptive method
  — effective
  — unrelated to coitus (especially as she will be newly married)
  — not masking menopause (an additional concern for women of her age)
  — little or no side effects
  — good control of cycle
  — protection against infections (especially if she has history of PID)
  — protection against gynaecological malignancies
  — protection against menopausal symptoms, osteoporosis and other effects of oestrogen deficiency.

85

- Effectiveness: most existing methods are effective. Sterilisation, IUCD, injectables and COC pills are particularly effective. Coitus interruptus, natural methods and spermicides are less effective.
- Relationship to coitus: barrier methods, coitus interruptus and spermicides are related to coitus. Natural methods restricts the days of intercourse. Other methods are not coitus-related.
- Masking menopause: progesterone-only pills (POP), COC pills and injectables might mask the menopause.
- Side effects: there are long lists of side effects of COC pills and IUCDs, which will not be repeated here. Mrs Lewis should be counselled about the common side effects.
- Control of cycle: COC pills offer good control of the cycle. Other contraceptives offer less good control.
- Protection against infections: barrier methods protect (but not completely) against infections. Spermicides, POP, injectables and COC pills might offer some protection. Other methods do not protect against infections, although the incidence of PID is actually lower with IUCD rather than higher, as commonly believed.
- Protection against gynaecological pathologies, menopausal symptoms, osteoporosis and other effects of oestrogen deficiency: levonorgestrel-releasing intrauterine systems offer endometrial protection for women on HRT. Other methods do not offer such protection.
- Written material given to Mrs Lewis. An immediate decision needs not be made in this consultation. Encourage her fiancé to attend for further discussion.

Simon, a 22-year-old intravenous drug addict, presented with two skin abscesses on the buttock. What immediate and future problems does he face?

CONSTRUCT

- Physical problems
  - — the skin abscesses, including secondary causes and complications
  - — local problems
  - — general and systemic health problems
  - — HIV and other infections
- Psychological problems
- Social problems.

ANSWER

Physical problems

The skin abscesses

- Complications: sinuses, fistulae, sepsis, septicaemia, complications of treatment (e.g. allergy to antibiotic, bleeding and local trauma from drainage procedure)
- Secondary causes: bacterial infection of perianal herpes, lymphogranuloma venereum, HIV infection, Crohn's disease.

Local problems

- Cellulitis, thrombophlebitis, skin abscesses, limb ischaemia.

General and systemic health problems

- Impaired local and general immunity, general constitutional weakness, fatigue
- Bacteraemia, septicaemia, endocarditis, bacterial and fungal pneumonia, septic pulmonary emboli, tuberculosis, hepatitis B and C, renal failure
- Respiratory: non-cardiac pulmonary oedema, aspiration, foreign-body embolisation, altered pulmonary function, asthma
- Gastrointestinal: mouth ulcers, nausea and vomiting, diarrhoea, constipation, abdominal pain
- CVS: chest pain, palpitation, dizziness
- CNS: confusion, convulsions, cognitive effects.

HIV and other infections

- Bloodborne infections: HIV, hepatitis B, C and D, syphilis, sepsis, septicaemia.
- Effects of drug use may be confused with symptoms of HIV infection. Heroin use and overdose may cause cough and dyspnoea. These can also be caused by *Pneumocystis carinii* pneumonia and tuberculosis. Confusion and convulsions related to heroin use may also be caused by CNS infections in HIV infection. Malnutrition in IVDU may cause sore mouth, gingivostomatitis and weight loss. Similar symptoms can also be caused by candidiasis, herpes infection, diarrhoea and CDC IV-A symptoms (constitutional symptoms defined as fever for more than 1 month, weight loss of more than 10% of baseline or diarrhoea for more than 1 month). Septicaemia and endocarditis caused by IVDU can also be caused by opportunistic infections and CDC IV-A symptoms.
- HIV infection does not progress more rapidly in IVDUs. However, bacterial pneumonia and tuberculosis are more common in IVDUs.

87

- There can be significant drug interactions in HIV-positive drug users. Methadone can lead to increased zidovudine (AZT) levels, whereas rifampicin and rifabutine can lead to decreased methadone levels.
- Many hepatologists are more conservative in treating hepatitis B and C in IVDU with alpha-interferon or lamivudine.

Psychological problems

- Depression, lack of self-esteem
- Psychosis and encephalopathy due to alcoholism and vitamin deficiencies
- Irritability and sleep disturbances due to drugs and withdrawal.

Social problems

- Alcoholism, abuse of other substances
- Poor living conditions, hygiene problems, relationship problems
- Financial problems, difficulty in securing a job
- Antisocial and criminal behaviour, prison sentences
- Unprotected sexual behaviour, STDs, poor uptake of contraception, unplanned and unwanted pregnancy of wife or girlfriend
- Problems in delivery of health care, poor attendance, poor compliance to treatment, difficult venous access for drug therapy
- Stigmatisation by GP, members of PHCT and others.

Mrs Miles, a 35-year-old secretary, was diagnosed by a surgeon as having early carcinoma of the breast. Breast-conserving lumpectomy was scheduled, but she was quite concerned about whether mastectomy would be a better treatment choice. What issues would you discuss with her?

CONSTRUCT

- Her knowledge of the disease
- Her attitude to the disease
- Her knowledge of the treatment options
- Her attitude and concerns about the treatment options
- Her health
  — physical
  — psychological
  — social
- Future roles of the GP and PHCT

ANSWER

Her knowledge of the disease

- How much does she know about carcinoma of the breast and the related factors?
- Does she have any of the risk factors?

Her attitude to the disease

- Has she ever blamed herself for causing the cancer (e.g. taking COC pills, not participating in a screening programme, taken certain foods, having 'bad genes')?
- Does she blame anyone else for causing the cancer?
- Can she accept the fact that she has cancer? Does she think that all cancers are incurable?

Her knowledge of treatment options

- How much does she know about the treatment options that are available? What explanations did the surgeon give her for the present course of management?
- What is her attitude to a mastectomy? Has she discussed this openly with her husband? What was her husband's reaction?
- She should be informed that in some circumstances breast-conserving surgery is possible for early cases. There has been no demonstrable difference in the rate of survival and risk of metastatic disease between women who have had a mastectomy and those who have had breast-conserving surgery, when the site and state of the tumour are such that the latter option is feasible.
- Radiotherapy after lumpectomy will further decrease the risk of local recurrence.
- Other methods to reduce the risk of recurrence, such as anti-oestrogen drugs (tamoxifen), multi-agent chemotherapy and ovarian ablation, are also available.
- She should be reassured that she has been referred to the proper specialist, and studies demonstrate that patients treated by specialists who treat many similar patients and have access to a full range of therapeutic options in a multidisciplinary setting have better outcomes.

- If possible, she might be given the option to obtain a second expert opinion.
- Suitable patient information leaflets on the treatment of early carcinoma of the breast can be given.

Her attitude and concerns about the treatment options

- Why is she worrying about going to have a lumpectomy? Are there any hidden worries? Are there any misconceptions? Does she know anyone with carcinoma of the breast? What treatment options did they have? What were the outcomes? Does she think that she would have the same outcome?
- What are her husband's attitude and concerns about the treatment options? Did he see the surgeon with her? Can he attend the surgery for further discussion?

Her health

Physical

- She must be physically prepared for the course of treatment. Any physical disease should be treated or controlled well.
- She is advised to have a normal, healthy lifestyle: a healthy diet, exercise, no smoking, no excessive alcohol intake, normal sex life.

Psychological

- Any anxiety? Depression? Sleep disturbances?
- Is she psychologically prepared for the course of treatment?

Social

- What is her recent relationship with her husband, her children, her boss and other people? Does she have good social support?
- How has her sex life been recently? Has the couple discussed their future sex life?
- Does she experience any difficulty in arranging sick leave for her treatment?
- Can she arrange for someone to help with her housework and caring for her children while she is away for treatment?
- Does she have any financial problems?

Future roles of the GP and the PHCT

- Providing continuous support and counselling
- Introduce her to local support groups
- Ensuring that she attends follow-up appointments and post-treatment mammography.

Mrs Johnson, aged 51 years, had been consulting you for abdominal distension for months. No objective sign was noted on abdominal and pelvic examinations. She was reassured that the distension was due to her irritable bowel. While you were on holiday, she was referred by your locum to the gynaecologist, and diagnosed as having carcinoma of the ovary. Describe your feelings and thoughts when you learn about the incident.

CONSTRUCT

- Negative ideas
- Neutral ideas
- Positive ideas.

ANSWER

Shock

- Initially I will be shocked as this is totally unexpected.

Denial

- Could there be a mistake? Are there two Mrs Johnsons on our list?

Guilt

- It must all be my fault. I should have referred her for an ultrasound earlier. I should not have gone on holiday.

Anger

- Why should this misfortune happen to me? Why did Mrs Johnson not tell me that the abdominal distension was different from her irritable bowel symptoms? Why did she not insist that something should be done?

Self-protection

- Other doctors would have behaved like me. After all you cannot just refer anyone with abdominal distension for ultrasound, can you?
- The outcome might not have been affected if she was referred earlier.
- I have always practised to a high professional standard.

Shame

- How can I face Mrs Johnson in the future?
- What will my partners and other practice staff think of me?
- What will the gynaecologist think of me?

Loss of confidence

- Is my history taking and physical examination technique that bad? My partners, the locum and other GPs are definitely better than me.
- Have I entered the wrong profession?

91

Depressed

- It is my own fault that the diagnosis was delayed. I am useless.
- I cannot improve my standard of care in the future (hopelessness), and no-one can help me (helplessness).

Relieved

- At least this is a good outcome. If I had not been on holiday, the diagnosis might have been even further delayed.

Acceptance

- The delay in diagnosis has happened. Nothing more can be done about it.
- I must look forwards. How can I prevent similar misfortunes again? Should I take more postgraduate courses? Should I join a Balint group? Should an audit be performed?

Jenny Adler 'kidnapped' her mother, 82-year-old Mrs Adler, and brought her to see you, as both Mr and Mrs Adler refused to seek help for Mrs Adler's dementia. Mr Adler insisted that the decline of his wife was a natural accompaniment of ageing.

1. Why might he deny the problem of his wife?
2. What investigations would you consider?
3. What ethical and legal considerations might you face in the long-term management?

CONSTRUCT

1. Reasons for denial

- Lack of knowledge
- Psychological denial
- Different time frame of observation
- Personal concealment and compensation
- Fear of labelling
- Feeling of guilt
- Fear of consequences
- Anticipated regret.

2. Investigations

- Tests to exclude common causes of dementia
- Tests to exclude alcoholism and substance abuse
- Tests to assess for cerebrovascular dementia
- Tests to exclude structural brain lesions
- Tests to assess nutritional state.

3. Ethical and legal considerations

- Consent to assessment and treatment
- Confidentiality
- Compulsory admission
- Access to medical records
- Conflict of interests
- Testamentary capacity
- Living will
- Euthanasia
- Abuse of the elderly.

ANSWER

1. Reasons for denial

There are several possibilities.

Lack of knowledge
Mr Adler may have a poor knowledge of dementia and the problems it causes. He may have known some relatives with much more severe dementia, and thus not realise that, although his wife's condition seems better than those others at present, she is in fact suffering from the same condition.

Psychological denial
Denial is a natural response to unfavourable messages. For some individuals, it is a necessary step towards understanding and acceptance.

Different time frame of observation
The GP sees Mrs Adler every few months and would notice an obvious deterioration in her intellect and memory. Jenny might see her every few weeks and notice some changes. Mr Adler, however, is living with her and sees her every day. As the changes are very subtle and gradual, it is understandable that he would not notice any change.

Personal concealment and compensation
Patients with early dementia tend to conceal their deficiencies and may even compensate by efforts in other mental areas not yet affected. For example, some patients might use a notebook to jot down all the necessary daily activities. It might not be obvious to other people that, without the notebook, the patient cannot even manage to prepare a meal.

Fear of labelling
Mr Adler may fear that his wife would be labelled as 'demented' or 'psychiatric', and thus isolated by other people.

Feeling of guilt
Mr Adler loves his wife, who has always been faithful to him. To complain about her problems might be seen by him as an act of disloyalty and lead to guilty feelings.

Fear of consequences
This is one of the most common reasons for late presentation of dementia. Mr Adler fears that should a diagnosis of dementia be made, his wife will be removed to an institution.

Anticipated regret
Some individuals may delay making decisions (such as to seek help) to avoid future regret. Others may make irrational choices based on incomplete evidence to avoid future regret.

2. Investigations

Investigations to rule out common causes of dementia include complete blood picture, ESR, renal function tests with electrolytes, fasting glucose (with or without an oral glucose tolerance test) and thyroid function tests (complete profile with free T_3, free T_4 and TSH).

Some practitioners might include the VDRL test, although generalised paralysis of the insane is a very rare cause of dementia now.

Parkinson's disease and parkinsonism are best detected by physical examination, not by investigations.

If alcohol and substance abuse cannot be ruled out by history, blood alcohol level, gamma-glutamyl transferase (gamma-GT) and serum and urine for toxicology screening might be needed. Medications as a cause of dementia should also be assessed by history and investigations if indicated.

As cerebrovascular dementia accounts for about 15% of cases in very old age groups, risk factors such as HT, smoking, hypercholesterolaemia, DM and atrial fibrillation should be assessed by history, physical examination and basic

investigations.

Structural lesions such as chronic subdural haematoma, primary and secondary cerebral tumours and normal pressure hydrocephalus are uncommon. If suspected clinically, contrast CT or MRI of the brain is indicated.

Demented patients are at risk of dietary deficiencies, and albumin, ferritin, B_{12} and folate levels may need to be measured depending on assessment and results of other investigations.

3. Ethical and legal considerations

The major ethical and legal considerations are outlined below.

Consent to assessment and treatment
Mrs Adler may not consent to assessment and treatment even after she has been given a detailed explanation of her condition. She has the right to refuse any intervention if she is capable of understanding and making the decision and if her behaviour does not pose risks to herself and other people.

Confidentiality
Information may need to be released to other health care workers such as the health visitor and the social worker. They also observe a code of confidentiality like medical practitioners.

Compulsory admission
In extreme conditions, compulsory admission might involve Mental Health Act Section 2 (admission for assessment), Section 3 (admission for treatment), Section 4 (emergency admission), Section 5 (holding power), Section 7 (guardianship) and National Assistance Act Section 47 (removal to a place of safety).

Access to medical records
Mrs Adler may demand access to her own medical records for a number of reasons. The Access to Health Records Act (1990) allow patients aged 16 years or over access to their medical notes, if written after 1 November 1990. However, the GP may withhold information if he believes that serious physical or mental harm will be incurred to the individual or others on the release of the information.

Conflict of interests
The interests of Mrs Adler, Mr Adler, Jenny, other family members and the GP may all be different and sometimes conflicts exist. Asking Jenny to attend her parents' house to do the housework daily may be welcomed by Mr and Mrs Adler, but unacceptable for Jenny.

The picture is more complicated if the practice is fundholding, as institutional and community resources are always limited.

Testamentary capacity
Mrs Adler may lose her testamentary capacity if she is 'incapable by reason of mental disorder of managing and administering her property and affairs'.

Living will
Mrs Adler might like to prepare a 'living will' directing that in the event of future incompetence to participate in a decision, active life-supporting measures should not be adopted. Such is to prevent prolonged unnecessary suffering related to heroic life-saving measures.

Euthanasia
'Passive euthanasia', the withdrawal of life-sustaining measures to allow a patient

95

to succumb to the disease, is different from 'active euthanasia', the deliberate administration of a lethal dose of a toxic substance. The latter is definitely illegal in the UK. But who should decide on when to withdraw active treatment? Should 'living wills' be legally binding? Is a case conference possible, or beneficial, in every case?

Abuse of the elderly

Demented patients are more liable to be abused. This is likely to be much underdiagnosed. To have a high index of suspicion is easier said than done. It is even more difficult to define 'emotional abuse', and the 'abusers' (carers) may be under as much stress as the victim.

Mrs Field, aged 39 years, consulted you in the sixth week of her first pregnancy about antenatal screening. She revealed that as she was a Roman Catholic she would keep the pregnancy even if the fetus had Down's syndrome. Upon your counselling, she decided that she would not undergo any of the investigations that aim to diagnose untreatable genetic and congenital conditions.

Three weeks later, you received the following letter:

10 June 1999
Dr XXX, Bonham Surgery
Dear Dr XXX

Mrs F Field, aged 39 years, attended our antenatal clinic yesterday. To our astonishment, she commented that she had been advised by you not to undergo screening for fetus chromosomal abnormalities.

You might have advised her on religious grounds. However, the costs and sufferings that a handicapped child can bring to the family should not be underestimated.

Upon our compassionate counselling, Mrs Field finally agreed to be scheduled for amniocentesis.

We believe that patients should be allowed to make decisions on their own, without undue influence or coercion. When they cannot come to a wise decision, they should be counselled by a specialist with expert knowledge in the field concerned.

Yours sincerely
YYY, FRCOG
Consultant Obstetrician

1. Describe your feelings on receiving the letter.
2. Mrs Green, aged 40 years, is also pregnant and consults you on similar issues. How would the incident with Mrs Field affect your counselling of Mrs Green?

CONSTRUCT

1. Reaction to letter

- Surprised
- Confused
- Annoyed
- Angry
- Curious
- Amazed
- Need for self-evaluation.

2. Counselling Mrs Green

- Be empathic, understand her concerns and expectations
- Be aware of negative feelings from last case, utilise lessons learnt from the previous case
- Early involvement of her husband
- Remind them of GP's role as counsellor, and of the need to make an informed choice themselves
- Maintain good relationship with obstetrician, understand what tests are being offered in the local centre

- Delay decision-making until the couple have seen the obstetrician if possible
- Respect the couple's decision
- Have clear documentation of process and results of counselling.

ANSWER

1. Reaction to letter

I was initially surprised when I received the letter as it was a highly unlikely outcome of the consultation.

I was also confused at why Mrs Field had changed her mind after a seemingly reasonable decision had been made based on her religious beliefs and the objective facts. Advice or information might have been given by the obstetrician. She might have discussed the situation with friends, or, more importantly, her husband, who might not be giving her unconditional support. Last, Mrs Field might fear that she would regret it later if amniocentesis was not performed, so-called anticipated regret.

However, Mrs Field might not have changed her mind at all. Her attitude was that she 'would not have any investigations aimed at diagnosing untreatable genetic and congenital conditions'. This is not necessarily incompatible with a decision to undergo amniocentesis.

I was also annoyed by the letter and felt intimidated and humiliated. As a GP, I seemed to have been reprimanded by the specialist and forced into a perpetuation of the teacher–student relationship. This also led to a loss of confidence, both generally as a GP and specifically as the counsellor and GP of Mrs Field.

I was angry, my anger being directed at Mrs Field who might have changed her mind, at the obstetrician for his misunderstanding my position as a responsible GP and an empathic and impartial counsellor, and at myself for having the misfortune to have counselled Mrs Field.

I was curious at why the obstetrician would think that it was I who advised her against antenatal screening, rather than that being her own decision. I was amazed by the 'compassionate counselling' offered to Mrs Field by staff of the antenatal clinic.

I also felt that there was a need for self-evaluation of my attitudes when counselling patients on issues with a strong moral or religious element, of my counselling skills and of my relationship with specialist colleagues.

2. Counselling Mrs Green

After the incident with Mrs Field, I would take a good history from Mrs Green should she consult me on the same issues. I would try to be empathic and understand her concerns and expectations from the consultation. I would try to understand, though not necessarily agree to, her moral and value ideas.

I would constantly remind myself that negative feelings from the previous case should not be brought to this case. Rather, the lessons learnt should be utilised to enhance this consultation.

I would try to involve her husband in the counselling process as early as possible, as the decision should be that of the family, and the later joys or regrets will be borne by the whole family.

I would ensure that Mr and Mrs Green understand my position as a counsellor and as their GP, and that my responsibility is to make them understand the issues and concepts involved in antenatal screening and to help them to reach an informed decision.

A good relationship with the obstetrician is vital in understanding what tests are being offered in the local hospital and what diseases such tests are aiming to diagnose. The GP should also understand whether the diagnosed conditions are potentially treatable or not.

The couple should be informed of the severity and significance of the conditions. The family may, for example, be able to accept a happy child with Down's syndrome, but not a child with spina bifida cystica, diplegia, faecal and urinary incontinence and hydrocephalus.

The risks of the procedures should be clearly explained, including risks of abortion, bleeding, infection and rhesus iso-immunisation.

Time should be given for the couple to digest the information. Several consultations may be needed to help them through this process.

They are encouraged to delay making a decision until they have discussed the issues with the obstetrician and among themselves privately. Whatever the decision is, it belongs to the couple and should be respected. The antenatal clinic and the obstetrician might be informed of the part played by the GP in the process.

Clear notes should be kept by the GP on the contents of the discussions with the couple. The GP should also constantly evaluate his interview and counselling technique, and familiarise himself with new developments in antenatal screening and diagnosis.

Andes and Martha have several years' history of recurrent genital herpes. Martha has never been pregnant and is planning to conceive. They are concerned about the effects of herpes on the pregnancy and the baby. How would you respond?

CONSTRUCT

- Understand concerns and expectations
- Review history
- Assess knowledge
- Explain risks of neonatal herpes: risk is likely to be small
- Explain prognosis of neonatal herpes: grave prognosis, but improving on treatment
- Measures to minimise the risk of neonatal herpes
- Pre-pregnancy counselling
- Sexual health.

ANSWER

Understand concerns and expectations

- What do they expect from the consultation?
- When are they planning to conceive?
- Do they have any other hidden worries or concerns?

Review history

- Medical, surgical, gynaecological, drug history, use of contraception, social history
- History of genital herpes: first symptomatic attack for both Andes and Martha, frequency and severity of subsequent attacks, any complications, use of antiviral agents (short-term and long-term prophylactic)
- History of other STDs and PID.

Assess knowledge

- How much do they understand about the cause of genital herpes, the role of antiviral agents, why there are relapses and remissions and the relationship of genital herpes to other STDs and to carcinoma of the cervix (no causal relationship)?
- How much do they know about effects of genital herpes on pregnancy, childbirth and the infant?

Explain risks of neonatal herpes

- Explanation should be given in nontechnical terms, at a level that they can understand and give feedback.
- Theoretically, herpes can be transmitted to the baby via the placenta (transplacental), during labour (intrapartum) and after delivery (postpartum).
- Transplacental transmission: risk is small, leads to early fetal death and spontaneous abortion.
- Intrapartum and postpartum transmission: can lead to neonatal herpes.
- Out of all the cases of neonatal herpes: about 5% are from transplacental transmission, 90% from intrapartum transmission and 5% from postpartum transmission. The implication is that most transmissions occur during labour.

- Risk of transmission: if mother has a primary attack during vaginal delivery, the risk of intrapartum transmission can be as high as 50%. If the mother is having a recurrent attack, the risk is only about 5%.
- If Andes and Martha only have one single strain of herpes virus (genital herpes can be from strains of both HSV-1 and HSV-2), Martha can only have a recurrent attack. The implication is therefore that the risk of transmission is low even if she is having an attack during pregnancy.
- The risk is even lower if HSV-2 antibody is present before pregnancy and if the partner is also seropositive. It has been said that the use of fetus scalp electrodes may increase the risk.

Explain prognosis of neonatal herpes

- Neonatal herpes: can be localised to the skin, eye and mouth (SEM syndrome), can affect the CNS and can disseminate to multiple organs (liver, lung, adrenal gland, brain, SEM). The implication is that it can be a serious disease.
- Prognosis of neonatal herpes (without antiviral treatment): death is uncommon for SEM involvement only, but 35–40% will have neurological problems. With encephalitis, the mortality is about 50%; with disseminated disease, the mortality is about 90%.
- With early diagnosis (by PCR) and antiviral treatment, a dramatic improvement in the prognosis is seen.

Measures to minimise the risk of neonatal herpes

- Martha should inform her obstetrician about her history of genital herpes.
- There is no fixed protocol to minimise risk. Some obstetricians screen weekly for viral shedding after the 36th week of pregnancy and consider elective low-segment caesarian section for those with viral shedding, unless the woman is already in labour and it has been more than 4 hours since membrane rupture.
- Other obstetricians are either more active or more passive in their intervention to prevent neonatal herpes.
- The couple should discuss measures to minimise the risk of neonatal herpes with their GP and their obstetrician again when Martha becomes pregnant.

Pre-pregnancy counselling

- This is a good opportunity to offer pre-pregnancy counselling on the physical and psychosocial preparations for the pregnancy.
- Areas covered: physical health, psychological health, social support, smoking, alcohol, diet, exercise, breastfeeding and finance.

Sexual health

- The presence of one STD indicates that the couple is at risk of other STDs and complications of STDs.
- Counselling on safe sex, barrier sex and STDs can be offered.
- Leaflets on genital herpes are given to those with herpes. The couple can also be introduced to the services offered by the Herpes Association.

CASE 42

Mrs Prince, aged 59 years, had Colles' fracture of the right forearm 2 weeks ago. She had surgical menopause at the age of 44 years and was put on HRT for some years.

1. What factors would you take into account in assessing whether she is at risk of osteoporosis? Which factors should be managed by the GP and which factors should be managed by specialists? Which factors are irreversible?
2. List your strategies in preventing osteoporosis for Mrs Prince.

CONSTRUCT

1. Risk factors

- General factors
- Lifestyle factors
- Medical factors.

2. Prevention strategies

- Primary prevention
- Secondary prevention
- Tertiary prevention.

ANSWER

1. Risk factors

General factors

- Family history of osteoporosis (irreversible)
- Early age of menopause, surgical menopause (HRT, given by GP generally)
- Low body weight (irreversible, unless specific factors exist).

Lifestyle factors

- Smoking (social support, counselling and control of withdrawal symptoms by GP)
- Alcohol (social support, alcoholics anonymous, treatment by GP/psychiatrist/clinical psychologist, treatment of complications by physician/hepatologist)
- Lack of exercise, or excessive exercise (advice by GP)
- Low calcium diet (advice to increase calcium intake by GP/dietitian)
- Compliance to treatment, HRT should be taken for at least 5–10 years for any demonstrable benefit (advice by GP).

Medical factors

- Oestrogen-deficiency states, length and compliance of HRT (given by GP)
- Corticosteroid-excessive states; primary, secondary or iatrogenic e.g. systemic steroids for frequent episodic asthma (best referred to endocrinologist)
- Thyroxin-excessive states; primary, secondary or iatrogenic (treated by GP, physician or endocrinologist)
- Malabsorptive states (best referred to a physician)
- Rheumatoid arthritis and other chronic rheumatology conditions (best referred to a physician or rheumatologist)

- Chronic liver and renal diseases (best referred to specialists)
- Any medical or psychosocial condition leading to prolonged immobilisation (treated by GP or appropriate specialists).

2. Prevention strategies

Primary preventive strategies
The aim of these strategies is to remove the causative agents or factors.

- active assessment and treatment of general, lifestyle and medical factors listed above
- no smoking, sensible alcohol intake (below 14 units per week for women)
- regular exercise
- skimmed milk or calcium replacements
- take medications only under medical advice.

Secondary preventive strategies
The aim of these strategies is to detect the disease at an early or asymptomatic stage.

- measuring hip, spine, or forearm body density by dual energy X-ray absorptiometry (DXA)
- spine bone density measurement by quantitative computerised tomography (QCT)
- forearm bone density measurement by single photon absorptiometry (SPA)
- ultrasound measurement of bone parameters (US).

At present, DXA and QCT are more widely used. The results of SPA and US are less standardised.
    These investigations should be performed in the following circumstances:

- when a fracture highly suggestive of osteoporosis has occurred, e.g. Colles' fracture as in Mrs Prince's case, or vertebral body or femoral neck fracture with minimal trauma
- when a medical condition predictive of osteoporosis is present, as listed above (depending on history and other assessment results)
- when Mrs Prince is already under treatment for osteoporosis (see below), to monitor the response.

Tertiary preventive strategies
The aim of these strategies is to prevent complications once a diagnosis is made, so as to decrease impairments, disabilities and handicaps.

- evaluate the present HRT of Mrs Prince
- give calcium supplements at 1 g/day
- consider other treatment options such as progestogens, biphosphonates, calcitriol, anabolic steroids, vitamin D and sodium fluoride
- consider referral to specialists
- monitor treatment clinically and with bone density scans
- education and environmental-modification to prevent falls
- referral to support groups and services for osteoporosis.

You are offering shared care for 57-year-old Mrs Bolton with atrial fibrillation and hypercholesterolaemia now on digoxin, warfarin and simvastatin. The target range of INR is 2.0–3.0. In the past month, her INR has shown high variability.

1. List the factors that may contribute to the high variability of her INR.
2. As a GP, what measures would you take to minimise the risk of haemorrhage?

CONSTRUCT

1. Contributing factors

- Psychosocial factors
  — incompliance in taking warfarin
  — incompliance in taking other medications
  — laboratory errors
- Physical factors
  — liver and renal diseases
  — other diseases
  — alcohol
  — other medications
  — diet.

2. Measures to minimise risk of haemorrhage

- Primary prevention
  — control above factors
  — arrangements for minor operations
  — arrangements for major operations
- Secondary and tertiary prevention
  — early detection and referral
- Practice protocol, audit and continued education
- Prevention of haemorrhage for others e.g. children.

ANSWER

1. Contributing factors

Psychosocial factors

- Incompliance in taking warfarin: this is the commonest correctable factor. Mrs Bolton should be requested to bring her tablets to the surgery so that the number of pills left can be assessed.
- Incompliance in taking other medications: the effect of warfarin is potentiated by HMG-CoA reductase inhibitors. Thus, whether simvastatin is regularly taken should be checked. It is important to ascertain whether Mrs Bolton is taking other medications unknown to the GP.
- Laboratory errors: any of the processes from blood taking, labelling, transportation of specimens, storage of specimens, testing, comparison with controls, printing reports and sending reports can go wrong. A common error is the acceptance of partially clotted blood by the laboratory.

Physical factors

- Liver and renal diseases: these lead to difficult control of the INR and increased risk of haemorrhage.

- Other diseases: anaemia, coexisting coagulopathy and malignancies may be factors.
- Alcohol: a significant change in the consumption of alcohol can be important.
- Other medications: medications that increase the INR include allopurinol, amiodarone, cephalosporins, cimetidine, erythromycin, metronidazole, omeprazole, quinidine, ranitidine and sulphonamides. Medications that decrease the INR include antacids, antihistamines, carbamazepine, penicillin, rifampicin and vitamin C.
- Diet: a large amount of vitamin K-containing green vegetables can significantly decrease the INR.

2. Measures to minimise risk of haemorrhage

The following measures help to minimise the risk of haemorrhage:

- The factor(s) leading to poor INR control must be identified and corrected.
- It must be stressed to Mrs Bolton that she must be very compliant in taking warfarin and other medications. All medications taken must be known to the GP. A family member can be appointed to help and support her in this aspect.
- Only fresh blood samples should be accepted by the laboratory so that the INR reported is reliable.
- Excessive alcohol consumption and sudden significant changes in alcohol consumption should be discouraged.
- For minor surgery or dental extraction, the warfarin should be reduced a few days before the operation. The target range on the day of surgery should be an INR of 1.5–2.0.
- For major operations, the anticoagulation is best adjusted by the physician. The target INR will be about 1.2 or less. When there is a high risk of thromboembolism, the patient can be switched to heparin and heparin stopped on the day of surgery.
- When there is unexpected haemorrhage with unidentifiable cause, or unexpectedly high INR results, the patient should be referred immediately to the care of the physician.
- A simple and clear information leaflet on anticoagulation can be given to patients and their families.
- Close communication should be maintained with the physician in the shared care programme.
- A practice protocol can be established for shared care with the physician for anticoagulation.
- There should be a practice system to call back defaulters.
- A plan of clinical audit and continued education for practice staff may also be beneficial.
- The risk of haemorrhage is not limited to the patients themselves. There should be precautions to prevent accidental self-poisoning by infants and children.

Mr Chan, a 46-year-old laboratory attendant, has a long history of asthma. Recently, he realised from the lay press that occupational exposure to urine of male rodents is a cause of asthma. He requests investigations to confirm this and a letter to his employer for insurance and compensation purposes. How would you handle this consultation?

CONSTRUCT

- History
  - his concerns and expectations
  - review history of asthma
  - his occupation
  - relationship of his symptoms with the exposure
- Examination
- Investigations
  - types of investigations available
  - indications and limitations
- Response to his request
- Review management of his asthma.

ANSWER

History

- His concerns and expectations: what recommendations does he expect in the letter? What long-term plans does he have for his occupation? How much does he know about the insurance policy?
- Review history of asthma: age at first onset? Frequency and severity of symptoms? Any seasonal change? Other differential diagnoses possible? Do the symptoms affect his work and hobbies? Has he been admitted to hospital for an asthma attack? What step of the BTS guidelines is he now on? Compliance to treatment?
- His occupation: detailed occupation history since he left school/college, including any temporary or unpaid voluntary work. Has he been exposed to laboratory animals, flour, grain dust (e.g. fungi, mites), enzymes (e.g. in biological detergents), formaldehyde, colophony, di-isocyanates, acid anhydrides or platinum salts?
- What does he suspect to be the major allergen?
- Are there any policies in his workplace to minimise such exposure? Does Mr Chan observe such policies?
- Are there any other workers in the same workplace with the same ailment?
- Temporal relationship of symptoms to exposure. In a typical case of occupational asthma
  - a known sensitising agent is present at work
  - the patient has been exposed to this agent for some time *before* the asthma develops
  - this sensitisation period can range from days to years
  - further exposure then brings about attacks, sometimes within minutes, but more often the attacks may *be delayed for hours* (it is thus typical for the patient to have symptoms in the evening or at night, *once he has left the workplace*)
  - the condition improves on holidays, especially long vacations.

Examination

- As for any other case of asthma include pre- and post-bronchodilator PFR measurements if possible to document reversibility of airway obstruction.

Investigations

- It should be explained to Mr Chan that relevant investigations include skin-prick tests, serial peak expiratory flow measurements, serology and bronchial provocation tests.
- However, not only are almost all these tests difficult to interpret, they are mostly performed by an occupational physician or a chest physician rather than by the GP.
- Moreover, bronchial provocation tests may potentially lead to severe acute attacks and anaphylactic shock, and must be performed in a hospital with full resuscitation facilities and supervised by an experienced physician.

Response to his request

- If the history of Mr Chan is definitely not indicative of occupational asthma, Mr Chan should be frankly informed so. If he insists that he does suffer from occupational asthma, referral for a second opinion should still be made.
- Otherwise, unless the GP or any of his partners has a special interest and expertise in occupational medicine and is actively engaged in such practice, it would be better for Mr Chan to be referred to an occupational physician for further assessment.

Review management of his asthma

- In the meantime, his asthma should be managed according to practice protocols or BTS protocols.

Eight-month-old Lucy was brought by her mother Mrs Young for routine screening for hearing deficit. There was no risk factor or special parental concern. The distraction test was to be done by you and Catherine, the practice nurse.

1. Describe how the distraction test is to be performed and the common pitfalls.
2. Describe how you would decode the following terms to Mrs Young, a secondary school teacher: false-negative result, sensitivity, positive predictive value, yield, incremental yield.

CONSTRUCT

1. Distraction test

- Arrangements for the test
  — the time and space
  — the partner
  — the room
  — the child
- The test
  — the distraction
  — the sound
  — other sources of stimuli
- Interpretation of result
  — criteria of a pass
  — declaration for a failure
- Other considerations
  — history taking
  — advice to parents
  — pathway for referral
  — audit
  — training for staff.

2. Decoding terms

- Decode in layman terms
- Give examples if relevant.

ANSWER

1. Distraction test

The distraction test must be performed with great care to minimise false-positive results that could lead to unnecessary anxiety and false-negative results that could lead to false assurance and delays in diagnosis and appropriate remedies.

Arrangements for the test

- The time and space: the test should be performed in protected time. The examination room should be quiet and free from disturbances.
  — pitfalls: performing the test in busy baby clinic, in a room with much background noise and with frequent disturbances by receptionists and telephone calls.
- The partner: the test is a job for two experts. Both the tester (the one in command) and the assistant should be well trained and preferably have performed the test together for some time. The tester (the GP) should be

distracting the child while the assistant (Catherine) should produce the sounds, not the other way round.
  — pitfalls: asking an untrained person (e.g. the Mrs Young) to be the assistant; the sound producer to be in command of the test rather than the distractor.
• The arrangement of the room: Lucy sits in the centre of the room, either alone or on her mother's lap. The GP sits behind a small table directly facing Lucy. Catherine produces sounds at two positions 45° behind Lucy. No other person should be in the room.
  — pitfall: any other arrangement.
• The child: the child should be 6–18 months old; it is best if the child is 6–9 months old. Lucy should be well and alert on the day of the test.
  — pitfalls: performing the test when Lucy is tired, irritable or has a febrile illness.

The test

• The distraction: a clearly visible moving toy is used. When Lucy's attention is being fixed on the toy, the movement is suddenly and quietly stopped, to be replaced by fine movements of the fingers of the distractor. At that instant (the plateau of attention), the sound is produced.
  — pitfall: poor timing due to lack of cooperation between the distractor and the assistant.
• The sound. five kinds of sounds can be produced: high-, medium- and low-pitch sounds from a single-pitch sound producer, human 'ss' and human 'hummm'. The sounds should be just audible.
  — pitfall: using cup-and-spoon, crumbling piece of paper or any other sounds or sounds that are too loud.
• Other sources of stimuli: there should be no other visual (eye movements of the distractor, shadows of the assistant), auditory (footsteps of the assistant), tactile (movements of Mrs Young) and olfactory (perfumes and body odours of the assistant) stimuli.
  — pitfall: other stimuli detected by the baby.

Interpretation of result

• Criteria of a pass: for each of the responses to high-, medium- and low-frequency sounds, a pass is attained if Lucy turns to the correct side on at least two out of the three times that sound is produced.
  — pitfall: producing a sound only once and declaring a pass.
• Declaration of a failure: if Lucy does not turn correctly for at least two out of the three times, she has failed the test for that frequency.
  — pitfall: testing repeatedly until she passes.

Other considerations

• History taking: the most sensitive method of detecting hearing loss is to ask the mother, rather than performing the distraction test.
• Advice to parents: Mrs Young should be informed that this is a screening test only and she should still pay attention to Lucy's development of hearing and speech.
• Pathway for referral: there should exist a predetermined smooth pathway for the referral of children who fail the distraction test i.e. test positive for a hearing abnormality.
• Audit: the uptake of the programme and outcomes of children who have tested positive for a hearing abnormality are good end-points for clinical audit.
• Training of staff: regular training and reviews are necessary.

2. Decoding terms

The result is *falsely negative* when the child in reality has an abnormality that the screening test fails to identify. For example, a child with a mild hearing impairment may pass a distraction test, the disability to be suspected only later by the parents and confirmed by an audiologist.

The *sensitivity* of a screening test is the ability of the test to pick up the abnormal children. For example, if there are 10 children who really have a hearing impairment and the test identifies 8 of them, the sensitivity of the test is 80%.

The *positive predictive value* of a test is the chance that a child really has an abnormality if the test result is positive. For example, if the test identifies 10 children who may have a hearing impairment, whereas only 7 are confirmed as having impaired hearing by the audiologist, the positive predictive value of the test is 70%.

The *yield* of a screening test is the proportion of children correctly picked up as having an abnormality. For example, if the distraction test is performed on 100 children, and 3 of them are correctly picked up as having a hearing impairment, the yield of the test is 3%.

The *incremental yield* of a new screening test is the additional proportion of children correctly identified as having an abnormality, as compared with an old test. For example, if both the old test and the new test are performed on 100 children, with the new test correctly identifying 10 children with a hearing impairment and the old test correctly identifying only 5, the incremental yield is 5%.

Jimmy, aged 18 years, has seven viral warts on his fingers and palms. He has tried salicylate ointment and plasters before and now requests 'more definite treatment' as the lesions interfere with his playing the cello. Describe your management.

CONSTRUCT

- History
  - concerns and expectations
  - past treatment
  - extent of disability
- Differential diagnosis – warts or callosities?
- Options of treatment and relative pros and cons
- Jimmy as equal partner in making an informed choice of treatment.

ANSWER

History

- Concerns and expectations: what does he mean by 'more definite treatment'? How much does he know about the modalities of treatment? Why does he turn up for more definite treatment here and now? Has there been any type of trigger event?
- Past treatment: form, extent and duration of all past treatments. Has he had any adverse reactions?
- Extent of disability: to what extent is his playing the cello affected? Is he a performance player? Is there a coming performance? (This is important as disability will increase in the first few days after invasive therapies, especially after cryotherapy.) Does he have any other disability? Do his warts affect activities of daily living? Does he swim? (If so, they may then spread to others.)

Differential diagnosis

- Are they really viral warts due to human papillomavirus? Can they be callosities? (Callosities almost invariably occur at sites of pressure. Warts can occur at sites of pressure as well as other palmar and plantar surfaces, and usually have a central darkened core. Moreover, severe callosities are rare except in heavy manual workers.)

Options of treatment

- Passive observation: spontaneous regression is related to the development of cell-mediated immunity. It may take 2–3 years. This might not be acceptable to the cellist.
- Keratolytic agents: Jimmy might not have been complying with the regime of applying keratolytic agents 2–3 times daily for the past few months. Some of these agents are messy and their effect is slow. The virus particles are not actually eradicated, and the lesions might relapse even though there is a temporary remission. (However, the same can also be said about the invasive therapies.)
- Surgical excision: ugly scars are likely to form. Surgery is reserved for large solitary lesions that fail to resolve by other methods.

111

- Electrocautery and electrodesiccation can give excellent cosmetic results under expert hands. Wound healing is usually fast and uncomplicated.
- Cryotherapy: this is increasingly becoming more popular. The final cosmetic result is unsurpassed under expert hands. Postoperative hyper- and hypopigmentation usually recovers spontaneously in months or years. However, there are postoperative blisters and even bullae which could prevent Jimmy from touching the cello for a week.
- Laser treatment: this achieves the best controlled tissue destruction. However, the apparatus and maintenance costs are astronomical. Laser treatment is usually reserved for facial warts on young female patients.

Jimmy as equal partner in making an informed choice of treatment

- Jimmy should be handled as an adult. The pros and cons of the different modalities of treatment should be presented to him so that he can make an informed choice. The GP might play an active advocacy role in the process.

Mrs Philips had been treated for panic disorder by your partner for 6 months. She saw you when your partner was on leave, disclosing for the first time that she had her attacks only in social situations when she was surrounded by unfamiliar people.

1. List your aims in your further history taking.
2. Speculate on the reasons why she disclosed this fact to you but not to your partner.

CONSTRUCT

1. Aims

- Understand ideas, concerns and expectations
- Development of doctor–patient relationship
- Ascertain diagnosis
- Assess severity and disability
- Assess social support
- Planning for treatment.

2. Reasons for her disclosure to you

- Reasons for her not disclosing the fact to the partner
- Reasons for her disclosing the fact to the new GP.

ANSWER

1. Aims

The aims in further history taking are:

- to understand why she turns up for the consultation here and now, her concerns, including hidden concerns, and her expectations from the consultation
- to initiate the development of a good doctor–patient relationship, which is a therapeutic tool for further interventions
- to elicit further symptoms to confirm the diagnosis of social phobia
- to assess the extent of the effects of social situations so as to differentiate between *generalised* social phobia and *discrete* (*circumscribed*) social phobia
- to assess for the severity of the social phobia and the disability caused i.e. the extent to which her life, her family, her career, her housework, her hobbies and her social activities are affected
- to understand her views on the causes and factors (predisposing, precipitating, perpetuating), nature, severity and treatability of her condition
- to evaluate whether she has other psychiatric problems, such as alcoholism, substance abuse, mood disorders, eating problems or sleep problems
- to assess her physical health
- to assess her sexual health
- to understand how her husband and family view her problems and to assess her social support
- to plan actively her treatment and rehabilitation e.g. to assess for contraindications to medications to be used.

2. Reasons for her disclosure to you

Reasons for Mrs Philips not informing her former GP

- 'This is absurd and irrational': one of the diagnostic criteria for social phobia (DSM-IV) is that the patient recognises that the fear is excessive and irrational. Thus, Mrs Philips views the problem as being absurd and unreasonable and would like to hide and conceal it.
- 'It will get better': she hopes that treatment for the panic disorder might also control her phobic symptoms.
- 'This is not a medically acceptable ticket to call for help': she would rather be treated for panic disorder and other psychosomatic problems than for social phobia.
- 'If he asks, I will tell him': should her symptoms be a common and recognised medical problem, the GP would have asked. (Social phobia is in fact the commonest anxiety disorder in the community. It is the third most common psychiatric disorder in developed countries, after depression and substance abuse.)
- 'I have known the GP for over 10 years...': a long 'mutual investment company' exists and any additional factor might upset the balance of the investments.
- 'Everyone will think that I am mad': Mrs Philips does not want to be labelled 'weak' or 'psychiatric' by the GP, her family and others.
- 'I will tell him if my fear does not improve by Christmas': denial and procrastination delay calling for help.
- 'I will tell him if I can no longer cope with my shopping': the tolerance limit has not been reached.

Reasons for Mrs Philips informing her new GP

- In general, the opposite of the possibilities outlined above are all feasible causes. Her problems might be getting worse, causing more disabilities and reaching her tolerance limit. She does not know the new GP well and a well established 'mutual investment company' is not yet formed.
- Her husband and family might have urged her to tell her GP.
- She might have read about social phobia in a magazine and changed her attitudes to the disorder.
- The simplest reason (which is *the* reason in this real case) is that the new GP asked her 'Are there any social situations you would avoid entering because of fear of humiliation or embarrassment?' *(In fact, Mrs Philips has been waiting for this question for 6 months.)*

Mr Davis, a 54-year-old businessman, complains of impotence for 3 months. Describe your approach to the management of Mr Davis.

CONSTRUCT

- Possible causes
  - physical
  - pharmacological
  - psychological
  - social
- History
- Physical examination
- Investigations
- Management
  - the dilemma – physical or psychological?
  - treat treatable causes
  - treat the couple, not the man alone
  - major modalities of treatment.

ANSWER

Possible causes

- Physical causes of impotence include structural, endocrine and other causes. The age of onset makes structural causes highly unlikely. Endocrine causes include DM, Cushing's syndrome, hypothyroidism and hypopituitarism. Only DM is common.
- Other physical causes include HT, peripheral vascular disease, cerebrovascular diseases and multiple sclerosis.
- Pharmacological causes are common. Alcohol, antihypertensives, antidepressants, antipsychotics and various hormones can all lead to impotence.
- Psychosocial causes interact with the physical causes. Anxiety, depression, stress, anger, guilt, a pressure to perform well and relationship problems may lead to and exacerbate impotence.

History

- The 'impotence': what does he mean by impotence? Onset? Progression? Any precipitating or perpetuating factor noticed? Any premature ejaculation? Any misconceptions? (The medical definition is actually the failure to initiate and to sustain an erection; it has nothing to do with ejaculation, amount of semen and quantitative and qualitative aspects of sperm.)
- The sex life: how is the couple affected? What are his wife's views on his impotence? Is she involved in any extramarital sexual activities? It is best if the couple can be interviewed together, with the prior consent of Mr Davis.
- His ideas about, concerns to do with and expectations from the consultation.
- Update his medical and surgical history, including psychological problems, travel history and use of drugs and alcohol.

Physical examination

- In the absence of any suspicion of specific causes, a general examination, including BP, chest, heart and abdomen is usually adequate. The external genitalia examination, including per rectal examination for prostate, might be added but is generally unrewarding.

- Doppler studies to assess for peripheral vascular diseases may be included.

Investigations

- In the absence of specific pointers, full blood count, ESR, fasting glucose, T_4, microurinalysis with or without ECG should be sufficient.

Management

- The dilemma – physical and psychological: whereas most physicians used to believe that as many as 90% of all cases of impotence were the result of psychological causes, evidence is accumulating that in many cases physical causes are underdiagnosed and undertreated.
- The extent of investigations to assess for physical causes and the threshold for referral thus depends on local resources and the practice policy.
- If a medical cause is found, the cause is treated or controlled. However, treating an apparent underlying cause may not lead to a complete recovery.
- It psychological causes are identified, depending on the chronicity and severity, referring the couple to a psychiatrist or clinical psychologist can be helpful. Some may have expertise in offering sex therapy and touching exercises, such as Master and Johnson's sensate focus programme.
- A referral to a urologist or genito-urinary physician with a special interest in impotence may also help. Some specialists give papaverine injections into the corpus cavernosum or prostaglandin E_1 injections. Some might advise on vacuum devices to help achieve an erection. The prospect of using viagra can also be discussed with Mr Davis.
- Accompanying problems such as failure to ejaculate or premature ejaculation should be managed. If the failure to ejaculate is related to sympathectomy, thioridazine or indoramin can be helpful. The squeeze technique applied by the woman before the moment of inevitable ejaculation may delay ejaculation. Clomipramine and serotonin-reuptake inhibitors are also helpful in premature ejaculation.
- With a logical management plan and a supportive empathic attitude from the GP and other health professionals, it is most likely that the couple will see an improvement and continue to enjoy a healthy sex life.

Sixty-year-old Mr Gray had stroke due to right middle cerebral artery occlusion 9 months ago. He now walks slowly but independently. He uses the right (dominant) arm rather than his left arm, the function loss of which being greater than expected from the neurological examination findings. He cares for himself with some assistance.

Mr Gray is living with his wife who is a secondary school teacher. He is now socially withdrawn and does not accompany Mrs Gray to church or other community activities. Mrs Gray, aged 52 years, is fit and healthy.

1. What factors may account for the discrepancy between the neurological deficit and loss of function of Mr Gray's left arm?
2. What areas of concern would you have for Mrs Gray?

CONSTRUCT

1. Factors related to loss of function

- Physical factors
  — dominance of right hand
  — sensory loss of left upper limb
  — apraxia
  — muscle wasting
  — joint contractures
- Psychosocial factors
  — lack of confidence
  — factors in the rehabilitation programme
  — self-neglect
  — secondary gains.

2. Concerns for Mrs Gray

- Physical health
- Psychological health
- Social health
- Other concerns.

ANSWER

1. Factors related to loss of function

Physical factors

- Dominance of right hand: as Mr Gray is right-handed and the left hand is now clumsy, he is naturally inclined to use his right hand more.
- Sensory loss of left upper limb: the neurological examination mainly detects the motor deficits, as the sensory deficits cannot be precisely documented and the dermatomes are overlapping. The sensory paresis is likely to be contributing to the functional loss.
- Apraxia: as the non-dominant parietal lobe is affected, sensory apraxia contributes to the functional deficit of the affected side.
- Muscle wasting: similar to disuse atrophy, muscle wasting occurs and is not limited to diseases causing lower motor neuron lesions.
- Joint contractures: mixed hypotonia and hypertonia can lead to joint contractures of the left arm, further contributing to the functional deficits.

117

Psychosocial factors

- Lack of confidence: any incident or misfortune such as falling and breaking a glass of water may render Mr Gray unwilling to use his left hand.
- Factors in the rehabilitation programme: Mr Gray might not be attending the physiotherapy and occupational therapy sessions compliantly, or might not find such sessions useful.
- Self-neglect: neglect of a limb is a well known consequence of apraxia and anosognosia.
- Secondary gains: consciously or subconsciously, Mr Gray may realise that not using the left upper limb reminds Mrs Gray and other people that he has had a stroke, and thus they are concerned about him and offer him assistance.

2. Concerns for Mrs Gray

Physical health

- Perimenopausal symptoms
- Risks of CVS and cerebrovascular diseases
- Risks of osteoporosis and the related complications
- Problems of the genito-urinary system
- Benefits and risks of HRT
- Physical stress and fatigue from teaching, housework and looking after Mr Gray.

Psychological health

- Any anxiety about the health of her husband?
- Any depression and sleep problems?
- Any 'empty nest' syndrome?
- Any plans and hopes for the future?
- Any hobbies, interests and pleasurable activities?

Social health

- Relating to her husband
  - how is her relationship with her husband?
  - can she cope with his physical and psychosocial deficits?
  - how well is she communicating with her husband?
  - how was their sex life before the CVA?
  - have they had sex since the CVA? If so, how often and have there been any difficulties?
  - has there been any personality change in her husband since the CVA? If so, has she been able to cope?
- Relating to other family members
  - how often did the couple see their children and/or grandchildren before the CVA? How often do they see them now?
  - does Mrs Gray need any assistance from other family members or relatives?
- Relating to other people
  - is she happy in her career as a teacher?
  - has she been seeing her friends more or less since her husband's CVA?
  - what is the extent of her social support network?
  - what support does she have from the PHCT and the GP?

Other concerns

- Any financial problems?
- Any potential medicolegal or ethical problems? Will? Living will?

Simon, aged 8 years, was referred to a paediatrician to assess his short stature. A diagnosis of constitutional delay in growth and puberty was made.

1. What features might have led the paediatrician to the diagnosis?
2. List the advantages and disadvantages of drafting a practice guideline for referrals related to growth and puberty.

CONSTRUCTS

1. Features leading to this diagnosis

- Features from the history
- Features from growth measurements
- Features from the physical examination
- Features from investigations
- Time factors.

2. Advantages and disadvantages of a practice guideline

- Advantages and disadvantages for the patients
- Advantages and disadvantages for the GPs, the practice and the paediatricians
- Other considerations.

ANSWER

1. Features leading to this diagnosis

Features from the history

- Family history of short stature
- Family history of growth delay
- Family history of delayed puberty.

Features from growth measurements

- Proportionate height, weight and HC
- Height, weight and HC not significantly below third percentile
- Height, weight and HC increasing along the percentile curves
- Normal growth velocity (from two measurements at least 3 months apart).

Features from the physical examination

- Proportionate height, weight and HC
- No dysmorphic features
- Normal trunk/limb proportions
- Normal or delayed pubertal staging
- No abnormal pubertal changes.

Features from investigations

- Normal or slightly delayed bone age (delayed bone age is a sign of *good* potential for future growth)
- Normal basic investigations results (which may include complete blood picture, fasting glucose, thyroid function test).

119

2. Advantages and disadvantages of a practice guideline

The use of practice guidelines in referrals related to growth and puberty:

Advantages	Disadvantages
Can assure early referrals for cases with reversible causes (protect the patients)	Even with the best guidelines, cases can still be missed
Guide doctors and other health professionals in their choice	Limit choice and flexibility, affects professional autonomy
Allow appropriate use of resources	No evidence that resources are wasted if decisions to refer are made on clinical judgement
Skeletons of guidelines already exist (e.g. Hall's reports)	Guidelines need time, manpower and expertise to set up
Local paediatrician or paediatric endocrinologist may be able to help	Different experts and authorities have different thresholds for referral
Guidelines are good educational tools for health professionals	Doctors may not think when they just follow the guidelines; the thinking process is educational
Clinical audits can be readily done if guidelines are followed	Audits are more important in areas with no fixed clinical guidelines
Guidelines can protect the GP from medicolegal consequences if they are drawn up along agreed principles and are followed	Faulty guidelines can lead to medicolegal consequences but who should then bear the responsibility?
The guidelines can include 'need to reassure parents' as an indication for referral, thus maximising flexibility	Every referral can then be justified as most parents would like to be reassured and this then makes the guidelines superfluous
This can be a precedent to establish and use guidelines in other areas of the child health promotion programme	More guidelines create more work for the GPs and health visitors
Guidelines should be used so that benefits and difficulties can be evaluated	No evidence that such guidelines are beneficial and risk-free in the long-term

LIST OF ABBREVIATIONS

ABC	airway, breathing and circulation	INR	international normalised ratio
ABPM	ambulatory blood pressure measurement	IUCD	intrauterine contraceptive device
AC	air conduction	IUGR	intrauterine growth retardation
AIDS	acquired immunodeficiency syndrome	IVDU	intravenous drug user
BC	bone conduction	KOH	potassium hydroxide
b.i.d.	twice a day	LDL	low density lipoprotein
BMI	body mass index	LOS	lower oesophageal sphincter
BP	blood pressure		
BTS	British Thoracic Society	MAOI	monoamine oxidase inhibitor
CBC	complete blood count		
CIN	cervical intraepithelial neoplasia	MMR	measles, mumps and rubella
CIS	carcinoma in-situ	MRI	magnetic resonance imaging
CLO	*Campylobacter*-like organism	NIDDM	non-insulin-dependent diabetes mellitus
CNS	central nervous system		
COC	combined oral contraceptive	NSAID	non-steroidal anti-inflammatory drug
COPD	chronic obstructive pulmonary disease	OG	obstetrics and gynaecology
CT	computerised tomography	OPD	outpatient department
CVA	cerebrovascular accident	PCR	polymerase chain reaction
CVS	cardiovascular system	PFR	peak flow rate
DBP	diastolic blood pressure	PHCT	primary health care team
DM	diabetes mellitus	PID	pelvic inflammatory disease
ECG	electrocardiogram	PMS	premenstrual syndrome
ENT	ear, nose and throat	p.r.n.	as required
ESR	erythrocyte sedimentary rate	QCA	quadricyclic antidepressant
GI	gastrointestinal	q.i.d.	four times a day
GP	general practitioner	RIMA	reversible inhibitor of monoamine oxidase
GUM	genito-urinary medicine	SARI	serotonin-2 antagonist/reuptake inhibitor
HAV IgG	hepatitis A immunoglobulin G		
HbA$_1$	glycosylated haemoglobin 1	SBP	systolic blood pressure
HbA$_{1c}$	glycosylated haemoglobin 1c	SLE	systemic lupus erythematosus
HBeAg	hepatitis B envelope antigen		
HC	head circumference	SNRI	serotonin noradrenalin reuptake inhibitor
HCG	human chorionic gonadotrophin	SSRI	selective serotonin reuptake inhibitor
HDL	high density lipoprotein		
Hib	*Haemophilus influenza* type b	STD	sexually transmitted disease
HIV	human immunodeficiency virus	T$_3$	triiodothyroine
		T$_4$	thyroxin-4
HMG-CoA	hydroxymethyl glutaryl coenzyme A	TCA	tricyclic antidepressant
		t.d.s.	three times a day
HPV	human papillomavirus	T/M	trichomonas and monilia
HRT	hormone replacement therapy	TSH	thyroid stimulating hormone
		UTI	urinary tract infection
HSV	herpes simplex virus	VDRL	Venereal Disease Research Laboratory
HT	hypertension		
IBS	irritable bowel syndrome	VLDL	very low density lipoprotein

MULTIPLE TRUE/FALSE QUESTIONS

Frozen shoulder:

1. conservative treatment is indicated for most cases
2. the diagnosis is usually made by contrast arthrography
3. there are three phases, each lasting 4–8 months
4. a differential diagnosis is adhesive capsulitis

A 13-year-old girl requests COC pills. She seems to understand the benefits and risks of taking oral contraceptives.

5. her mother should be informed against the wishes of the girl
6. the GP commits an offence legally if he prescribes
7. the GP commits an offence legally if he refuses to prescribe
8. the GP breaches his terms of service if he prescribes

Cervical polyps

9. may be malignant
10. may extend to the vulva
11. are soft and bright red
12. are very common
13. can be safely removed by the GP in his surgery

Vasomotor rhinitis

14. typically worsens on exercise
15. may be caused by cardiac failure
16. is typically worse on lying down
17. is worse after alcohol
18. commonly coexists with allergic rhinitis

According to the Mental Health Act (1993)

19. signatures of two doctors are needed for admission under section 2, usually a GP and a psychiatrist
20. section 4 is emergency admission by signature of any one doctor for up to 72 hours
21. section 2 is admission for assessment by the nearest relative or approved social worker
22. section 3 is admission for treatment for up to 2 years

Atrial fibrillation can be caused by

23. hypertension
24. sinoatrial disease
25. alcoholic cardiomyopathy
26. pulmonary embolism
27. lobar pneumonia

All patients initially diagnosed to have hypertension should have

28. 24-hour urine for catecholamines
29. chest X-ray
30. urinary cortisol
31. microurinalysis
32. ultrasound of the kidneys

The Standing Medical Advisory Committee recommendations for antibiotic prescribing in primary care are

33. antibiotics should never be prescribed over the telephone
34. no antibiotic should be prescribed for viral pharyngitis
35. the course of antibiotics for uncomplicated cystitis in women should be limited to 7 days
36. no antibiotic should be prescribed for simple coughs and colds
37. no antibiotic should be prescribed for uncomplicated otitis media in children

In the stepwise approach to manage chronic asthma

38. the GP should start on step 1 and gradually step-up
39. the GP should start on steps 4 or 5 and gradually step-down
40. peak flow rates should be monitored for all patients
41. step 4 is inhaled beta-2 agonist when required with high-dose inhaled steroid regularly
42. step 4 is regular inhaled steroid with regular inhaled bronchodilator

Endometrial carcinoma:

43. multiparity is a predisposing factor
44. DM is a predisposing factor
45. early menopause is a predisposing factor
46. ovarian tumours can be a cause

Hypertensive retinopathy:

47. 'silver wiring' suggests at least grade 1 retinopathy
48. is a good indicator of damages to the arterioles in other parts of the body
49. 'soft exudates' are believed to be real exudates
50. 'hard exudates' are white deposits of lipids
51. flame-shaped haemorrhages suggest at least grade 2 retinopathy

Contraindications to the MMR vaccine include

52. congenital adrenal hyperplasia on glucocorticoid and mineralcorticoid replacements
53. pregnancy
54. history of egg allergy
55. history of allergy to neomycin
56. untreated malignant disease

The following are transmissible by sexual contact:

57. hepatitis A
58. hepatitis B
59. hepatitis C
60. hepatitis D
61. hepatitis E

Common causes of acute lower GI bleeding in adults are

62. colorectal carcinoma
63. diverticular disease
64. Meckel's diverticulum
65. haemorrhoids
66. polyps

Posterior dislocation of shoulder:

67. is a common sequelae after a convulsion
68. the diagnosis is frequently missed in a lateral film
69. a direct blow to the front of shoulder can be a cause
70. is less common than anterior dislocation

Gallstones:

71. only about 50% of individuals with gallstones have symptoms
72. the associated pain is mostly in the right upper quadrant
73. intolerance of fatty food is not a symptom
74. dyspepsia itself is not an indication for surgery
75. carcinoma of the gall bladder is present in most patients with gallstones

Virtually all participants taking an MSc course in general practice agreed that the course

76. increased the GP's understanding of patients' beliefs and behaviour
77. enabled the GP to provide a better quality of care to patients
78. enabled the GP to be more critical of his own work and that of others
79. increased the GP's confidence as a teacher
80. helped the GP to implement good practice

Monitoring for adult DM patients should always include

81. microalbuminuria
82. HbA_1
83. Doppler ultrasonography
84. supine and standing BP
85. visual acuity

Causes of pruritus ani in adults include

86. haemorrhoids
87. lichen planus
88. psoriasis
89. *Enterobius vermicularis* infestation
90. IBS

Chondrodermatitis chronica helicis

91. often involves the external ear canal
92. usually affects adolescents and young adults
93. is histologically related to squamous cell carcinoma
94. is typically painless
95. commonly ulcerates

Globus hystericus:

96. the discomfort is usually exacerbated by eating
97. it is a diagnosis made by exclusion
98. it may be related to cricopharyngeal spasm
99. a course of amitriptyline usually helps
100. the presence of dysphagia casts doubt on the diagnosis

Giving oestrogen alone as HRT is likely to increase the risks of

101. breast tumour
102. ovary tumour
103. cervix tumour
104. endometrial tumour

Acute leukaemia may manifest with

105. purpura
106. 'flu-like' symptoms
107. sore throat
108. cervical lymphadenopathy
109. herpes labialis

Child benefit

110. can be claimed by blood relatives only
111. continues until the child reaches the age of 16 years
112. has a low uptake
113. is contributory

The cervical smear screening programme:

114. yearly screening is not significantly better than 3-yearly screening
115. all women of reproductive age should be screened
116. it is a primary preventive strategy for cervical carcinoma
117. the smear can be taken by the practice nurse
118. yearly screening is necessary for some patients

Gout

119. usually affects one joint at a time
120. is nearly always present with hyperuricaemia
121. is mostly due to increased production of uric acid
122. developing at an early age suggests secondary causes
123. is significantly related to obesity

Atopic eczema is associated with

124. allergic colitis
125. allergic rhinitis
126. lactose intolerance
127. atopic urticaria
128. Down's syndrome

Secondary tumours in bones:

129. most breast secondaries are osteoblastic
130. most are osteoblastic
131. virtually all are visible on plain X-ray films
132. prostatic secondaries are commonly osteolytic

Substance abuse:

133. short-acting benzodiazepines more commonly lead to dependence than long-acting benzodiazepines
134. tolerance and withdrawal symptoms are common for cannabis use
135. physical dependence is unusual for amphetamine abuse
136. sudden barbituate withdrawal commonly leads to convulsions
137. cocaine is the commonest illegal drug taken in the UK

Primary prevention of rabies:

138. active immunisation of possible contacts
139. passive immunisation of possible contacts
140. killing stray dogs
141. vaccinating domestic dogs
142. animal quarantine

Routine seminal analysis

143. can be done on a sample of semen in a condom ejaculated at intercourse
144. cannot replace the postcoital test
145. should be performed after normal levels of sexual activity for 2 days
146. include tests for anti-sperm antibodies

Fractured scaphoid:

147. surgical intervention is frequently indicated
148. the usual cause is a fall on the dorsiflexed hand
149. surgery is indicated for fractured scaphoid tubercle
150. marked displacement of the fragments is characteristic

Possible indications for emergency tracheostomy:

151. laryngeal foreign body
152. diphtheria
153. laryngeal web
154. acute epiglottitis
155. subglottic stenosis

Acute frontal sinusitis:

156. orbital cellulitis is an important complication
157. amoxycillin with metronidazole is a good treatment of choice
158. radiological signs are commonly seen
159. cluster headache is an important differential diagnosis
160. pain is typically worse at night

The rheumatoid hand:

161. ulnar deviation of the fingers is typical
162. the swan-neck deformity is a flexion deformity of the proximal interphalangeal (PIP) joint
163. Z-deformity of the little finger is characteristic
164. boutonnière deformity is hyperextension of the PIP joint and flexion of the distal interphalangeal joint

The penicillins:

165. their dose need not be modified in patients with renal failure
166. cloxacillin is superior to flucloxacillin as the absorption of the former is better
167. clavulanic acid alone has no antibacterial activity
168. salbactam is a beta-lactamase inhibitor
169. a rash is seen in 20–30% of all patients with infective mononucleosis given ampicillin

Complications of uterine fibroids:

170. fatty change may render the fibroids radio-opaque
171. hyaline degeneration is a process of aseptic necrosis
172. sarcomatous change is rare
173. red degeneration is usually painless
174. cystic change is a sequel to hyaline degeneration
175. torsion of subserous pedicles is painful

Protective factors for Alzheimer's disease:

176. aluminium exposure
177. female sex
178. high educational level
179. smoking
180. HRT

Breath sounds are

181. vesicular with prolonged expiration in acute bronchitis
182. high-pitched bronchial in collapse due to obstruction of the major bronchus
183. harsh vesicular in pleural effusion
184. high-pitched bronchial in lobar pneumonia
185. bronchial in asthma

Menière's disease:

186. vertigo is usually persistent
187. intramuscular chlorpromazine is helpful in an acute attack
188. age of onset is usually in the fourth or fifth decades
189. it is bilateral in most cases
190. labyrinthectomy is usually effective in restoring the hearing

For rubella

191. the incubation period is about 10–14 days
192. the risk of congenital infection in the first 4 weeks of pregnancy is as high as 80%
193. suboccipital lymph nodes are typically tender
194. pneumonitis is the commonest complication
195. the rash typically affects the trunk first

According to the Access to Health Records Act 1990

196. there is no right of access to records written before November 1991
197. access is not limited to computer-held records
198. no fee can be charged for record access
199. records of the PHCT are exempt from patient access
200. the GP has 7 days to respond to a request for record access

Important factors that cause peptic ulcer are

201. NSAIDs
202. diet
203. *Helicobacter pylori* infection
204. alcohol
205. smoking

Rinne's test:

206. if AC is greater than BC, the test result is negative
207. if AC is greater than BC on the left side, the hearing of the left ear is normal
208. if AC is less than BC on both sides, one can safely conclude that there is conductive hearing loss in both ears
209. a 256 Hz tuning fork should be used
210. if AC is just equal to BC, a conclusion that there is no conductive hearing loss can still not be drawn

Urethral caruncle

211. is a whitish chalky mass
212. is typically tender
213. is usually posterior to the urethral meatus
214. commonly occurs in adolescents
215. causes deep dyspareunia

Reflux oesophagitis:

216. reflux occurs because the resting pressure of the lower oesophageal sphincter is increased
217. the lower oesophageal sphincter is normally situated above the diaphragm
218. clearance of acid from the oesophagus to the stomach is enhanced in the supine position
219. patients who have undergone a vagotomy cannot have reflux oesophagitis
220. 24-hour pH monitoring is important in the management of reflux in many infants

Urinary incontinence in women:

221. most cases are caused by detrusor instability
222. surgery has an important role in stress incontinence
223. most consider their work affected
224. most consider their social life affected
225. oestrogen may help in stress incontinence

Causes of acute stridor in a child aged 30 months:

226. laryngomalacia
227. croup
228. diphtheria
229. angioneurotic oedema
230. foreign body

Storage, distribution and disposal of vaccines:

231. vaccines should not be accepted if more than 24 hours have elapsed since they were posted
232. refrigerators should be defrosted regularly
233. incineration is not a recommended method for disposal of unused vaccines
234. frozen ice packs should be in contact with the vaccine to ensure that the required temperature is maintained during transportation
235. unused portions of multi-dose vials must be discarded after the session

Rotator cuff lesions:

236. degeneration is almost always a prerequisite for a tear
237. most tears start at the subscapularis tendon
238. frozen shoulder is the usual sequel to a complete tear
239. in a complete tear of the supraspinatus, the joint communicates with the subacromial bursa

A child with an ear grommet inserted

240. may need repeated operations if effusion recurs
241. is not allowed to swim
242. is expected to have abnormal impedance tympanometry results
243. should have the grommet removed under local anaesthesia after 6 months
244. should have regular hearing tests

Foreign bodies in the external auditory meatus:

245. general anaesthesia may be needed in an uncooperative child
246. live insects can be killed by olive oil
247. syringing is usually unrewarding
248. the most important complication is otitis externa
249. treatment is within the competence of the GP in most cases

Symptoms of endometriosis:

250. pain on defaecation
251. haematuria
252. rebound tenderness of the abdomen
253. intestinal obstruction
254. dysuria
255. pain in mid-cycle

Thiazides may cause

256. hyperuricaemia
257. hypoglycaemia
258. hyperlipidaemia
259. hypersensitivity
260. thrombocytopenia

Patients removed by GPs from their lists:

261. unreasonable requests for home visits is not a common cause for removal
262. higher rates of removal are noted for children under 5 years and young women
263. violent behaviour is a common cause for removal
264. such removal is permissible by the 1990 contract and the 1991 fundholding scheme
265. unreasonable requests for medication is a common cause of removal

Urinary calculi:

266. calcium phosphate stones are commonest in the UK
267. renal colic usually causes intermittent pain changing every few minutes
268. probenicid is indicated for uric acid stones
269. bendrofluazide reduces urinary calcium excretion
270. allopurinol helps in treating calcium oxalate stones

Management of suspected ectopic pregnancy:

271. there is an increased risk of recurrence of ectopic pregnancy if the tube is conserved
272. a pregnancy test is often helpful
273. ultrasound is of limited use
274. blood transfusion is frequently needed

Hallux valgus is

275. commoner in males
276. the commonest foot deformity in adults
277. commonly painful
278. often familial
279. not familial when it occurs in adolescents

Important causative factors of acne include

280. bacteria
281. food
282. hormones
283. heredity
284. inflammation

Dietary management in adults with DM:

285. the nutritional content and distribution of the daily food intake should be kept constant
286. the proportion of carbohydrates should be between 30–40%
287. soluble fibre-rich foods are highly recommended
288. the total energy intake daily should always be specified
289. alcohol intake should be forbidden

Ectopic pregnancy:

290. the incidence is higher in the black population
291. congenital malformations of the uterus and the fallopian tubes are the commonest predisposing factor
292. IUCD is a predisposing factor
293. the incidence is about 1 in 2000 in the UK
294. endometriosis is a predisposing factor
295. the HCG level is usually sky high

Hypochondriasis:

296. it is a somatisation of internal psychological distress
297. the sufferers are not malingering
298. delusional parasitosis is a common example
299. Munchausen's syndrome is a common example
300. dermatitis artefacta is a common example

The Census:

301. long-term illness is included in the survey
302. it is carried out every 10 years
303. household amenities are included in the survey
304. the data is treated in the strictest confidence

Cardiac murmurs:

305. not all innocent murmurs extend into the diastolic phase
306. the murmur in mitral stenosis is localised at the apex
307. early diastolic murmur at the heart apex suggests aortic or pulmonary regurgitation
308. ejection systolic murmur at the heart base suggests aortic stenosis or pulmonary stenosis
309. pansystolic murmurs can only be caused by mitral regurgitation, tricuspid regurgitation or ventricular septal defect

The National Curriculum Council recommended that the following components should be emphasised in health education:

310. sex education
311. substance use and abuse
312. nutrition
313. exercise
314. family life education
315. psychological health

Users of COC pills have an increased risk of

316. pulmonary embolism
317. ovarian cancer
318. cerebrovascular disease
319. endometrial cancer
320. venous thromboembolism

133

Atrophic vaginitis

321. causes a pink discharge
322. causes deep dyspareunia
323. usually does not respond to local oestrogen
324. is related to lack of oestrogens
325. may need antibiotics

Age of puberty:

326. a girl with no menses at 14 years of age should be investigated
327. usually no cause is found for a girl with menarche at 9 years of age
328. usually a cause is found for a girl with thelarche at 6 years of age
329. isolated adrenarche should always be investigated

EXTENDED MATCHING QUESTIONS

Option list

(A) chloroquine toxicity
(B) digoxin toxicity
(C) glaucoma
(D) lens dislocation
(E) migraine
(F) retinal haemorrhage
(G) retinitis pigmentosa
(H) optic chiasma lesion
(I) transient ischaemic attack
(J) vitreous opacities

Instruction

For each patient with visual complaint, select the single most likely diagnosis. Each option can be used once, more than once, or not at all.

Items

330. A 29-year-old man has double vision in one eye.
331. A 78-year-old man presents with transient acute spontaneous loss of vision in one eye.
332. A 23-year-old woman sees lightning flashes and a 'wavy' appearance of the environment.
333. A 49-year-old man complains of floaters of dusts and spots.
334. A 68-year-old woman presents with transient acute spontaneous loss of vision of both eyes.
335. A 75-year-old man presents with sudden onset of curtain drawn over one eye.
336. A 9-year-old boy has ataxic neuropathy and loss of night vision.
337. A 16-year-old child with delayed onset of puberty has loss of lateral vision in both eyes.
338. A 65-year-old woman complains of halos around lights.
339. A 45-year-old woman complains of yellow vision.

Option list

(A) ankylosing spondylitis
(B) gouty arthritis
(C) osteoarthritis
(D) osteochondritis dissecans
(E) Perthes' disease
(F) polymyalgia rheumatica
(G) pseudogout
(H) psoriatic arthropathy
(I) Reiter's disease
(J) rheumatoid arthritis
(K) septic arthritis
(L) SLE

Instruction

For each patient with joint problem, select the single most likely diagnosis. Each option can be used once, more than once, or not at all.

Items

340. A 28-year-old man has painful knees and ankles and a rash on his glans penis. He has history of urothritis due to *Chlamydia trachomatis*.

341. A 26-year-old medical student has pain and stiffness of the lower back for 6 months. Examination reveals pain over the bilateral sacroiliac joints.

342. A 68-year-old woman with DM has fever and severe pain in her right knee for 1 day. She has chills, rigor and appears confused.

343. A 67-year-old man complains of severe pain and stiffness in the muscles of the shoulder and pelvis for 3 weeks, particularly early in the morning. He has malaise and his ESR is elevated.

344. A 45-year-old woman has insidious onset of pain affecting the distal joints of the upper limbs symmetrically. She has weight loss. Examination revealed tender and swollen interphalangeal joints with slight deformities.

345. A 60-year-old man wakes up with severe pain in the metatarsal-phalangeal joint of his left big toe. The joint is red, swollen and tender and the overlying skin is shiny.

346. An 18-year-old football player has a swollen left knee, which gives way for 3 months. Examination reveals quadriceps wasting and tenderness in the lateral aspect of the joint.

347. An 18-year-old female patient has symmetrical joint pain affecting distal limb joints with early morning stiffness. She is being treated for a photosensitive dermatitis on the face.

1. **True**

2. **False**
   The diagnosis is usually made clinically. A plain X-ray may be needed to exclude other structural lesions.

3. **True**
   The freezing stage of increasing pain and stiffness, the frozen stage of persistent stiffness, and the thawing stage of gradual return of mobility.

4. **False**
   Frozen shoulder means adhesive capsulitis.

5. **False**

6. **False**

7. **False**

8. **False**

9. **True**

10. **True**

11. **True**

12. **True**

13. **False**
    Hysteroscopy, then dilatation and curettage are needed to assess for and treat other polyps higher up and other associated pathologies.

14. **False**
    Improves after exercise.

15. **True**

16. **True**

17. **True**

18. **True**

19. **True**

20. **True**

21. **True**

22. **False**
    6 months.

23. **True**

24. **True**

25. **True**

26. **True**

27. **True**

28. **False**
    Only if history suggests pheochromocytoma.

29. True
For cardiomegaly, signs of heart failure and rib notching in coarctation.

30. False
24-hour urine for cortisol only if Cushing's syndrome is suspected.

31. True
For proteinuria, glycosuria and proteinuria.

32. False
Only if renal diseases are suspected.

33. False
Should be prescribed only in exceptional circumstances.

34. True

35. False
3 days.

36. True

37. False
No formal recommendation.

38. False
Start on the most appropriate step and adjust either up or down.

39. False

40. False
Not feasible for some, e.g. small children.

41. False
Step 1: occasional inhaled beta-2 agonist
Step 2: step 1 + regular low-dose inhaled steroid or regular inhaled histamine-release inhibitor (cromoglycate)
Step 3: step 1 + regular high-dose inhaled steroid
Step 4: regular high-dose inhaled steroid + regular inhaled beta-2 agonist
Step 5: Step 4 + regular oral steroid.

42. False

43. False
Nulliparity is a predisposing factor.

44. True

45. False
Late menopause.

46. True
If they secrete oestrogens.

47. True

48. True

49. False
Believed to be microinfarcts.

50. True

51. False
At least grade 3.

52. False
Any replacement hormones and topical steroids are not contraindications.

53. True

54. False

55. True
The vaccine contains neomycin and kanamycin.

56. True

57. True
By oral–anal contact in homosexuals and heterosexuals.

58. True

59. True
Although the risk is probably lower than for hepatitis B.

60. False
Theoretically possible as the routes of transmission are similar to those for hepatitis B. Moreover, it is a deficient virus and always coexists with hepatitis B. However, no documented case of sexual transmission has been reported as yet.

61. False
Theoretically possible as the routes of transmission are similar to those for hepatitis A. However, there is no documented case of transmission by sexual contact.

62. False
Important but uncommon.

63. True

64. False
Rare.

65. True

66. False
Rare.

67. False
It may occur after a convulsion, but is uncommon.

68. False
The diagnosis is frequently missed in an anteroposterior film. Thus meticulous clinical examination and a lateral film are necessary.

69. True

70. True

71. False
Only 10% have any symptoms or signs.

72. **False**
Pain is mostly felt in the epigastrium.

73. **True**

74. **True**
Dyspepsia is not a symptom of uncomplicated gallstones.

75. **False**
Gallstones are present in most patients with carcinoma of the gall bladder.

76. **True**

77. **False**

78. **True**

79. **True**

80. **False**

81. **True**

82. **True**

83. **False**
Not of much use, as DM mainly affects the small vessels and significant foot problems can occur with a normal ankle–brachial index.

84. **True**
For postural hypotension caused by autonomic neuropathy.

85. **True**

86. **True**

87. **True**

88. **True**

89. **True**
Threadworm.

90. **True**

91. **False**
Usually affects rim of helix only.

92. **False**
The elderly.

93. **False**
Unrelated, but resembles this carcinoma morphologically.

94. **False**
Usually painful.

95. **True**

96. **False**
Relieved by eating.

97. **True**

98. **True**

99. **True**
Helps in most psychosomatic conditions.

100. **True**

101. **True**

102. **False**

103. **False**

104. **True**

105. **True**
HIV infection, syphilis, SLE and leukaemia are among the diseases that can present in almost any manner.

106. **True**

107. **True**

108. **True**

109. **True**

110. **False**
Can be claimed by the legal guardian living with the child.

111. **False**
Until the age of 18 years if the adolescent is in full time secondary education.

112. **False**
Uptake is high.

113. **False**
Noncontributory.

114. **True**
Yearly screening detects about 93% of all cases whereas 3-yearly screening detects about 91%. Thus the increase is only marginal.

115. **False**
Only those who have had sexual activity.

116. **False**
Secondary.

117. **True**

118. **True**
For women with a history of abnormal smear, with genital warts, with evidence of HPV infection, or whose partners have genital warts.

119. **True**

120. **False**
The two are related but different conditions. Gout sufferers need not have high levels of urate, and individuals with hyperuricaemia might not have gout.

121. **False**
   In most patients it is related to a genetically determined tendency of decreased uric acid excretion.

122. **True**

123. **True**

124. **True**
   Especially in cow's milk protein intolerance.

125. **True**
   Also asthma and allergic conjunctivitis.

126. **False**
   Cow's milk protein intolerance only. Lactase deficiency is either autosomal recessive of young onset in Caucasians, or autosomal dominant of older onset in non-Caucasians.

127. **True**

128. **True**

129. **False**
   Most are osteolytic.

130. **False**
   Most are osteolytic.

131. **False**
   Many are revealed only by isotopic bone scans.

132. **False**
   Osteoblastic.

133. **True**
   Contrary to common belief.

134. **False**
   Uncommon.

135. **True**

136. **True**

137. **False**
   Most believe that cannabis is the commonest.

138. **True**
   With diploid cell strain vaccine.

139. **True**
   With human rabies immunoglobulin.

140. **True**

141. **True**

142. **True**

143. **False**
   Collection is by masturbation unless this is impossible for the man concerned. Spermicides are present in most condoms.

144. True

145. False
Specimen should be collected after abstinence from sexual activities, including masturbation, for 3–5 days.

146. False
These are produced by the female.

147. False
Most are reducible under anaesthesia.

148. True

149. False
Conservative management.

150. False
Little or no displacement.

151. True

152. True

153. False
A chronic condition.

154. True

155. False
A chronic condition.

156. True
In children, caused by *Haemophilus influenzae* type b before 1992, *Staphylococcus aureus* after 1992 when universal Hib vaccination was introduced.

157. True
Should cover most organisms.

158. True
Opacity or fluid level.

159. True
Bilateral periodic frontal headache with nasal congestion in male adolescents, termed cluster migraine in the past.

160. False
Worse at midday.

161. True

162. False
The described is boutonnière deformity.

163. False
Z-deformity commonly occurs in the thumb.

164. False
The described is swan-neck deformity.

165. False
They can accumulate, leading to encephalopathy.

166. False
Flucloxacillin is almost twice as well absorbed.

167. False
It itself is a beta-lactam, although its antibacterial activity is weak. It is a potent beta-lactamase inhibitor.

168. True
Unasyn is ampicillin with salbactam.

169. False
If the diagnosis is true, as many as 90% will develop a rash.

170. True
Because of calcification.

171. True

172. True

173. False
Painful.

174. True

175. True

176. False
Suspected to be a risk factor.

177. False
Females are more prone.

178. True

179. True

180. True

181. True

182. False
Diminished or absent breath sounds.

183. False
Diminished or absent.

184. True

185. False
Vesicular with prolonged expiration.

186. False
Intermittent.

187. True

188. True

189. False
About 25% of all cases.

190. **False**
Mainly for relief of the vertigo.

191. **False**
16–21 days.

192. **True**

193. **True**

194. **False**
Arthralgia is the commonest complication. Pneumonitis is a complication of measles and chicken pox.

195. **False**
The rash typically appears first behind the ears and on the forehead.

196. **True**

197. **True**

198. **False**

199. **False**

200. **False**
21 days.

201. **True**

202. **False**

203. **True**

204. **False**

205. **True**

206. **False**
Positive. The interpretation is that there is no significant conductive hearing loss. The patient can thus be
- normal
- have very mild conductive hearing loss (e.g. incomplete blockage by wax)
- have sensorineural hearing loss of mild or moderate severity (if the sensorineural hearing loss is very severe, BC will be greater than AC as BC is heard by the opposite ear).

207. **False**

208. **True**
However, sensorineural hearing loss can still not be excluded.

209. **False**
512 Hz. Lower frequencies are for testing vibration sensation.

210. **True**
When AC = BC, the following possibilities apply:
- normal, the patient is not very sensitive to intensity of sounds
- very slight conductive hearing loss
- sensorineural hearing loss of mild or moderate severity.

211. **False**
Bright red fleshy mass.

212. **True**

213. **True**

214. **False**
Perimenopausal.

215. **False**
Superficial dyspareunia.

216. **False**
The resting sphincter pressure is decreased, while the number of transient relaxations is increased.

217. **False**
Below the diaphragm.

218. **False**
Clearance is impaired in the supine position.

219. **False**
The pancreatic enzymes and unconjugated bile salts can still be offending agents.

220. **True**
It documents the severity and frequency of reflux and guides treatment.

221. **False**
Detrusor instability (urge incontinence) alone accounts for about 10%; 85% have stress incontinence alone. The rest have either true incontinence (e.g. caused by a fistula), overflow incontinence (e.g. caused by a neuropathic bladder) or a combination of types.

222. **True**

223. **True**

224. **True**

225. **False**
In urge incontinence.

226. **False**
Chronic stridor, rare after 1 year of age.

227. **True**

228. **True**

229. **True**

230. **True**

231. **False**
48 hours.

232. **True**
With care that the temperature of the vaccine does not fall outside the specified range during the period.

233. False
Either heat inactivation or incineration can be used.

234. False
These cause the vaccine to freeze.

235. True

236. True

237. False
Supraspinatus tendon.

238. False
Almost never. It follows a partial tear only.

239. True

240. True
Further drainage and reinsertion of grommet.

241. False
Controversial, but most ENT surgeons would allow swimming but not diving.

242. True

243. False
Would extrude spontaneously.

244. True

245. True

246. True
Then syringing.

247. False
Usually successful.

248. False
Iatrogenic trauma is the most important complication.

249. True

250. True
Endometriosis can affect almost every organ in the pelvis and the lower abdomen.

251. True

252. False
Rebound tenderness is possible on rupture or impending rupture of a chocolate cyst. However, this is a sign and not a symptom.

253. True

254. True

255. True
Ovulation pain is common for normal women and especially severe for women with endometriosis.

256. **True**

257. **False**
Hyperglycaemia, worsening DM control.

258. **True**

259. **True**

260. **True**

261. **False**
An important cause.

262. **True**

263. **True**

264. **True**

265. **True**
Mainly for addictive drugs.

266. **False**
Calcium oxalate.

267. **False**
Pain is usually constant during attacks.

268. **False**
Contraindicated as it is uricosuric. Allopurinol as xanthine oxidase inhibitor helps.

269. **True**

270. **True**

271. **True**

272. **True**

273. **False**
The tubal mass may not be visible. However, a coexisting intrauterine pregnancy and blood in the pouch of Douglas can be excluded.

274. **True**

275. **False**
Commoner in middle-aged and elderly women.

276. **True**

277. **False**
Most are painless unless there are complications such as inflamed bunion or secondary osteoarthritis.

278. **True**

279. **False**
Strongly familial in adolescent sufferers.

280. **True**
Propionobacterium acnes.

147

281. **False**
Much evidence of lack of association.

282. **True**
Increased sensitivity to androgens.

283. **True**
Often familial.

284. **True**
Roles of inflammatory cells and cytokines.

285. **True**

286. **False**
Carbohydrate 50–60%, protein 10–15%, fat 30–35%.

287. **True**

288. **False**
Unmeasured DM diet is recommended for relatively mild cases not on insulin and not on oral hypoglycaemic agents.

289. **False**
As long as the caloric intake is taken into account and the safety limits are not exceeded.

290. **True**

291. **False**
PID is the commonest predisposing factor.

292. **False**
IUCDs have a protective effect against ectopic pregnancy. However, they have an even higher protective effect against normal pregnancy. Thus, the overall incidence of ectopic pregnancy is decreased. However, if a woman becomes pregnant with an IUCD in situ, the probability of the pregnancy being ectopic is higher than in other women with no IUCD.

293. **False**
About 1 in 200.

294. **True**
If there are chocolate cysts in the tubes.

295. **False**
HCG is indicative of molar pregnancy. A molar pregnancy can, however, also be ectopic and has a high HCG level.

296. **False**
It is a morbid preoccupation with serious medical diseases.

297. **True**

298. **False**
Uncommon.

299. **False**
Those with Munchausen's syndrome believe that they do not have a disease.

300. **False**

301. True

302. True

303. True

304. False
Collective data is available by various means. Individual answers are treated in the strictest confidence.

305. False
The systolic vibratory murmur, commonest innocent murmur in childhood, does not extend into the diastolic phase; the pulmonary flow murmur also does not extend into the diastolic phase. The venous hum is continuous; it commonly extends into diastole.

306. True

307. False
Early diastolic murmur at the heart base.

308. True
Or aortic or pulmonary flow murmurs.

309. True
Generally true, except for shunt murmurs with very soft diastolic components taken as pansystolic.

310. True
It is just common sense that all should be emphasised.

311. True

312. True

313. True

314. True

315. True

316. True

317. False
Protective effect.

318. True

319. False
Protective effect.

320. True

321. True

322. False
Superficial dyspareunia. Deep dyspareunia suggests cervicitis, PID, IUCD in younger age groups, or retroverted uterus.

323. False

324. True

149

325. True
To treat secondary infections.

326. False
Not unless there are other problems.

327. True
Usually no cause even at younger ages. For boys with premature onset of puberty, a cause is usually found.

328. True

329. False

330. D

331. I
The attack involves circulation to the retina.

332. E

333. J

334. I
The attack involves circulation to the visual pathways or the occipital lobes.

335. F

336. G
He has abetalipoproteinaemia.

337. H

338. C

339. B

340. I
The rash is circinate balanitis. The eyes, palms and soles should also be examined.

341. A

342. K

343. F

344. J

345. B

346. D

347. L

MULTIPLE TRUE/FALSE QUESTIONS

Exogenous eczemas include

1. discoid eczema
2. allergic irritant dermatitis
3. asteatotic eczema
4. pompholyx
5. atopic eczema

A good screening test should fulfill the following criteria:

6. treatment for the condition must be available
7. the case finding should be a continuous process and not a 'once and for all' project
8. the test must be acceptable to the population concerned
9. the positive and negative predictive values should approach 100%
10. the sensitivity and specificity should approach 100%

Contraindications for HRT include

11. history of endometrial adenocarcinoma
12. migraine on combined hormone tablets
13. history of ovarian cancer
14. severe GI upset on combined hormone tablets
15. little or no menopausal symptoms
16. family history of thromboembolism

First rank symptoms of schizophrenia:

17. passivity is the feeling of emotions or movements being controlled by another person or an external object.
18. thought insertion is inserting one's thoughts into another person
19. thought echoing is speaking one's thoughts out aloud
20. thought withdrawal is the experience of one's thoughts being taken away
21. almost all patients with schizophrenia have at least one first rank symptom in the acute stage

Posterior dislocation of the hip:

22. concomitant fracture of the acetabular roof is common
23. it is commoner than anterior dislocation
24. the sufferer is a pedestrian in a car accident in most cases
25. the leg appears shortened, adducted and externally rotated

IBS:

26. an age of onset at 20–40 years is typical
27. dyspepsia is part of the syndrome for many sufferers
28. the radiological appearance is usually diagnostic
29. it remains a diagnosis by exclusion
30. small doses of amitriptyline are frequently helpful

Causes of neutropenia:

31. miliary tuberculosis
32. Crohn's disease
33. typhoid fever
34. viral hepatitis
35. hypothyroidism

Booking intervals:

36. longer consultations are associated with less stress for doctors
37. fewer antibiotics would be prescribed with longer consultations
38. most doctors would have liked longer booking intervals
39. the extent of dealing with psychosocial problems is not significantly changed with longer consultations
40. most doctors do not think that longer intervals would result in a higher standard of care

Uterine adenomyosis:

41. the endometrial glands usually do not menstruate
42. diffuse enlargement of the uterus is characteristic
43. dysmenorrhoea is characteristic
44. absence of pseudocapsules is characteristic

Ear syringing:

45. either sodium bicarbonate or normal saline should be used
46. ceruminolytic agents are documented to be superior to water in the softening of wax
47. every GP should be able to perform this
48. perforated tympanic membrane is a contraindication
49. a sterile technique is unimportant

Salivary calculi:

50. they rarely cause swelling of the salivary glands
51. removal of intraductal stones under local anaesthesia is possible
52. most occur in the submandibular gland
53. they are not usually palpable
54. they are mostly radio-opaque

Signs of aortic regurgitation:

55. collapse pulse
56. bounding pulse
57. soft mid-systolic murmur
58. capillary pulsation in nail folds
59. femoral bruit

The Court Report (1976) of the Committee on the Child Health Services recommended that

60. district handicap teams should be established
61. the child health service should be increasingly oriented to prevention
62. sex education should be made compulsory against the wishes of the parents
63. at least one Consultant Community Paediatrician should be appointed in every district

Risk factors of COPD include

64. atmospheric pollution
65. occupational fumes and dusts
66. smoking
67. alpha-1-antitripsin deficiency
68. protease inhibitor phenotype of MM

The following actions may be considered as serious professional misconduct by the General Medical Council:

69. testing blood for HIV antibody without the informed consent of a patient
70. informing the PHCT that a patient is HIV positive without the informed consent of the patient
71. refusing to take necessary blood samples from an HIV-positive patient
72. informing the regulatory authorities that a colleague is HIV positive

Causes of constant vertigo:

73. Menière's disease
74. migraine
75. cardiovascular diseases
76. posterior fossa tumour
77. benign positional vertigo

Recommended therapies for cervical ectropion:

78. no treatment
79. electrocautery
80. laser cauterisation
81. cryotherapy
82. deep electrocauterisation

Salmonellosis:

83. salmonellosis is typically caused by *Salmonella enteritidis* or *S. typhimurium*
84. salmonellosis is usually treated with cefuroxime or cefotaxime
85. anti-diarrhoeal agents should not be prescribed for salmonellosis
86. the rash in typhoid fever typically appears on the seventh day
87. the Widal reaction is still considered the most reliable test for the enteric fevers

Suicide cases:

88. frequent GP consultations is an established risk factor
89. only 30% have consulted their GP in the preceding 6 months
90. about 80% are men
91. alcohol abuse is a risk factor
92. men are more likely to have history of mental illness in the preceding year

CIN:

93. CIN I corresponds to CIS
94. it is caused by human herpesvirus type 2
95. the diagnosis of moderate dysplasia is made on cervical smear
96. sufferers should be informed that they have early cancer of the cervix
97. no treatment may be necessary in some cases

Uterine fibroids:

98. are rarely found below the age of 30 years
99. become smaller in pregnancy
100. become larger at menopause
101. arise in the endometrium
102. are commoner in nulliparous women
103. may cause irregular menstruation

Fracture-dislocation of the upper forearm (Monteggia):

104. the upper third of the radius is fractured
105. close reduction is usually the treatment of choice for adults
106. pulling up a child forcefully is the usual cause
107. the ulnar head is dislocated

Treatment of ovarian tumours:

108. the role of a second-look laparotomy is controversial
109. an attempt should be made to conserve the greater omentum
110. surgical removal is usually necessary
111. the presence of ascites indicates malignant tumour with intraperitoneal
     spread
112. chemotherapy has little role
113. radiotherapy has little role

Otitis externa:

114. pain is typically increased by jaw movements
115. it can be a presenting sign of HIV infection
116. discharge is usually profuse
117. meticulous aural toilet is the core of treatment
118. increased sweating in hot climates is a predisposing factor

Salpingitis:

119. treatment should be commenced after high vaginal swab is taken
120. some cases are due to *Trichomonas vaginalis* infection
121. most patients should be admitted
122. most cases of recurrent infections are the result of inadequate use of antibiotics
123. an IUCD is a predisposing factor
124. contact tracing is necessary for many cases

After myocardial infarction

125. many patients can be discharged in 5–7 days
126. many patients drive again in 4–6 weeks
127. about 10% of all patients die within the first month
128. poor ventricular function and arrhythmias are indicators of poor prognosis
129. old age is associated with a higher mortality

Disability living allowance:

130. has two components
131. is mutually exclusive to most other benefits
132. was previously known as the invalid care allowance
133. is noncontributory

Functional dyspepsia is characterised by

134. pain unaffected by antacids
135. pain exacerbated by food
136. vomiting leading to immediate relief of pain
137. nocturnal pain
138. improvement on eradication therapy for *Helicobacter pylori*

The following oral glucose tolerance test results are diagnostic of DM:

139. venous plasma glucose of 11.4 mmol/L, fasting
140. whole blood glucose of 7.0 mmol/L, fasting
141. venous plasma glucose of 7.0 mmol/L, fasting
142. venous plasma glucose of 8.9 mmol/L, 2 hours after glucose load
143. whole blood glucose of 8.8 mmol/L, 2 hours after glucose load

Tennis elbow:

144. the origin of the elbow extensors is affected
145. prolonged tennis playing is the commonest cause
146. the medial epicondyle is affected
147. sudden major injury is a typical factor
148. entrapment of a branch of the ulnar nerve is believed to be a cause in some cases

HT

149. is defined as the BP above the normal level for the population
150. increases complications in a linear fashion
151. should always be treated only after at least three BP measurements at suitable intervals
152. should always be treated by nonpharmacological methods first
153. is a target for primary, secondary and tertiary prevention

Signs of an unruptured ectopic pregnancy:

154. abdominal guarding and rebound tenderness
155. blood oozing from the external cervical os
156. swelling on one side of the uterus
157. hypotension and tachycardia

Obsessive compulsive disorder:

158. obsessions with rituals are more resistant to treatment than obsessions without rituals
159. the sufferer hates the obsession and the compulsion
160. psychotherapy is the first line of management for most sufferers
161. genetic factors are important
162. SSRIs have been shown to be of benefit

Pharyngeal pouches

163. often cause dysphagia
164. are usually anterior to the oesophagus
165. commonly cause neck swellings
166. are commonly seen in young adults
167. commonly cause a gurgling sound

Differential diagnoses of a single scaly lesion on the upper arm of an 18-year-old individual:

168. pityriasis rosea
169. psoriasis
170. dermatophyte infection
171. herald patch
172. discoid eczema

Heartsink patients

173. have a lower referral rate than other patients
174. are mostly women
175. typically present with a list of problems
176. usually have more psychosocial problems than other patients

Oral hypoglycaemic agents:

177. glibenclamide is considered a high-potency second-generation sulphonylurea
178. extra-pancreatic effects have been demonstrated
179. they should not be used with insulin together
180. tolbutamide is relatively long acting
181. glibenclamide is notable for its proneness to cause hypoglycaemia in the elderly

Ruptured Achilles tendon:

182. incomplete tear is commoner than complete tear
183. most patients are over 40 years of age
184. the commonest complication is shortening of the tendon
185. a gap is usually not visible
186. it is usually accompanied by a tear of the soleus muscle

Women with recurrent UTIs are recommended to

187. empty their bladder regularly
188. increase fluid intake
189. take antibiotics only if an infection is documented
190. douche after sexual intercourse
191. bathe in a bubble bath

HIV-positive individuals should not receive the following vaccines:

192. BCG
193. tetanus
194. measles
195. yellow fever
196. live typhoid

A 30-month-old girl presents with a 2-day history of unilateral bloodstained nasal discharge. The likely diagnosis is

197. vasomotor rhinitis
198. foreign body
199. nasal trauma
200. nonaccidental injury
201. acute sinusitis

Tuning fork tests:

202. the tests can be used in children above the age of 6 years
203. if the Rinne test is positive on both sides and the Weber test is central, the hearing of the patient must be normal
204. the Weber test is mainly used to differentiate between conductive hearing loss and sensorineural hearing loss
205. they can be replaced by the pure tone audiogram if this is available in the practice
206. they can be replaced by tympanometry if this is available in the practice

Chronic pancreatitis:

207. cholelithiasis is the commonest cause in the UK
208. acute pancreatitis rarely proceeds to chronic pancreatitis
209. exocrine and endocrine disturbances are common
210. proton pump inhibitors preserve the activity of pancreatic extracts
211. DM should be managed with insulin

Common reasons for GPs deviating from their own rules of good practice:

212. clinical uncertainty
213. ignorance of principles of good practice
214. lack of time
215. fear of litigation
216. patient demand

***Trichomonas vaginalis* infestation:**

217. the partner should always be treated
218. it does not infest the cervix
219. it is sexually transmitted unless proven otherwise
220. treatment is with local clotrimazole
221. diagnosis is best made on wet film examination

Useful signs to distinguish bacterial from viral sore throat:

222. colour of tonsillar exudate
223. inflammed irregular pharyngeal mucosa
224. high fever
225. tender cervical lymph nodes
226. presence of tonsillar exudate

Risk factors for Alzheimer's disease:

227. male sex
228. smoking
229. high educational levels
230. Down's syndrome
231. head injury
232. NSAIDs

Nasopharyngeal carcinoma

233. is screened by X-rays of the nasopharynx
234. is aetiologically related to cytomegalovirus
235. causes early local symptoms
236. is most common in the Indian subcontinent
237. is mainly treated by complete excision

Human specific immunoglobulins are available for

238. hepatitis C
239. rabies
240. measles
241. chicken pox
242. adenovirus

Antibiotics significantly modify the clinical outcome in

243. sinusitis
244. tonsillitis
245. acute otitis media
246. acute bronchitis
247. pharyngitis

Fractured shaft of humerus:

248. the weight of the arm is usually adequate to achieve reduction
249. the radial nerve may be damaged
250. a spiral fracture usually heals in 2 weeks
251. a spiral fracture is usually caused by fall on the hand

Vulval swellings:

252. condylomata lata are noninfectious gummas in tertiary syphilis
253. carbuncles are painful lumps
254. condylomata acuminata are viral warts caused by HPV
255. molluscum contagiosum are caused by HSV infection
256. Bartholin's abscess should be treated by excision

Useful clinical features indicating the chronicity of a patient with allergic rhinitis:

257. violent sneezing
258. Dennie–Morgan folds
259. watery rhinorrhoea
260. excessive lacrimation
261. hay fever salute

Section 47 of the National Assistance Act (Removal to place of safety):

262. a place of safety is usually a geriatric or psychiatric ward
263. it is not applicable to cases of self-neglect
264. application can be initiated by the GP
265. it should be likely that the health of the patient will substantially improve upon such removal

The aminoglycosides:

266. oral streptomycin is effective against tuberculosis
267. the dose of gentamicin depends on renal function
268. topical neomycin is given for infections of the eye and skin
269. all are nephrotoxic and ototoxic
270. all are mainly excreted by the kidneys

Recurrent dislocation of the patella:

271. it is diagnosed by the apprehension test
272. weakness of the vastus lateralis is an important factor
273. dislocation is always to the lateral side
274. genu valgum can be a contributing factor

Sinus rhythms:

275. sinus bradycardia occurs in normal people during sleep
276. acute symptomatic sinus bradycardia can be treated with intravenous atropine
277. verapamil is a cause of sinus tachycardia
278. pulsus paradoxicus is a sinus rhythm
279. pulsus paradoxicus is useful in assessing the severity of asthma

The following should alert the GP to the diagnosis of bronchial carcinoma:

280. pleural effusion
281. irregular well circumscribed pulmonary opacity
282. elevation of a hemidiaphragm
283. unilateral hilar enlargement
284. lobar or segmental collapse

Antibiotics for respiratory tract infections:

285. the prescription of antibiotics is unrelated to whether psychosocial issues are explored
286. the severity of tympanic membrane changes is a good indicator of subsequent clinical course in otitis media in children
287. antibiotics are likely to be of marginal benefit for pharyngitis and otitis media
288. patients with lower respiratory tract symptoms more often ascribe their symptoms to infections
289. the predictive value of clinical findings in most respiratory infections is low.

The ^{13}C-urea breath test for _Helicobacter pylori_

290. diagnoses active infection
291. is not recommended as a test of cure
292. has high sensitivity and low specificity
293. is generally more useful than serology
294. requires sophisticated equipment to collect the samples

Ruptured biceps tendon:

295. the belly of the muscle is usually too high
296. the patient is usually over 50 years of age
297. good muscle function usually returns spontaneously
298. osteophytes in osteoarthritis of the shoulder are likely to play an important part

Alcoholic liver disease includes the following:

299. cholestasis
300. fatty liver
301. hepatocellular carcinoma
302. hepatitis
303. cirrhosis

Obesity

304. is commoner in lower socioeconomic groups
305. is an early feature in Prader–Willi syndrome
306. has a strong familial component
307. may lead to Perthes' disease, Blount's disease and slipped femoral epiphyses
308. is usually accompanied by decreased insulin levels

Transdermal patches of HRT:

309. skin reactions are common
310. the major disadvantage is limited absorption of hormones through the skin
311. compliance is usually better than oral therapy
312. it is pharmacokinetically inferior to oral tablets

The Manchester operation for vaginal prolapse comprises

313. shortening of the cardinal ligaments
314. anterior colporrhaphy
315. posterior colporrhaphy
316. amputation of the cervix

Neck pain:

317. aggravation by coughing or sneezing suggests raised intracranial pressure
318. most resolves in 1 week
319. blood tests are often helpful
320. referral to occipital region suggests pathology in the posterior fossa
321. paraesthesia and muscle weakness suggest radiculopathy

Under the Education Act 1986

322. the content of sex education for children with moderate learning difficulties should be different
323. parents should be informed about and involved in school sex education
324. parents have a legal right to refuse sex education for their children
325. parents can raise concerns about school sex education in annual parents' meetings

161

EXTENDED MATCHING QUESTIONS

Option list

(A) autosomal dominant (not triplet repeat)
(B) autosomal dominant (with triplet repeat)
(C) autosomal recessive
(D) chromosomal
(E) mitochondrial
(F) non-genetic
(G) X-linked dominant
(H) X-linked recessive

Instruction

For each patient with genetic disease, select the single most likely diagnosis. Each option can be used once, more than once, or not at all.

Items

326. Duchenne muscular dystrophy
327. tuberous sclerosis
328. neurofibromatosis type 1
329. myotonic dystrophy
330. ovarian agenesis
331. haemophilia B
332. Wilson's disease
333. Sturge–Weber syndrome
334. phenylketonuria

Option list

(A) acute angle closure glaucoma
(B) acute iritis (anterior uveitis)
(C) allergic conjunctivitis
(D) bacterial conjunctivitis
(E) corneal abrasion
(F) episcleritis
(G) foreign body
(H) herpes simplex corneal ulceration
(I) posterior uveitis
(J) Sicca syndrome
(K) subconjunctival haemorrhage
(L) viral conjunctivitis

Instruction

For each patient with red eye(s), select the single most likely diagnosis. Each option can be used once, more than once, or not at all.

Items

335. A 9-year-old girl with atopic eczema complains of itchy red eyes with watery discharge.
336. A 25-year-old man with ankylosing spondylosis complains of red eyes for 2 days with purulent discharge. Vessel dilatation is diffuse. Pupils are normal in size. Vision is normal.
337. A 35-year-old woman presents with bilateral painful eyes for 3 days. Vessel dilatation is mainly around cornea. Pupils are small. Visual acuity is mildly decreased.
338. A 68-year-old woman presents with sudden onset of reddened right eye. She has no pain. A patch of haemorrhage is seen.
339. A 38-year-old housewife complains of red and painful left eye for 1 day. Examination reveals purulent discharge and normal-sized pupils.
340. A 56-year-old man presents with very painful right eye and seeing halos. The right pupil is fixed and dilated.
341. A 40-year-old man presents with bilateral painful red eyes. Blood vessels are most prominent temporally.
342. A 35-year-old woman presents with mildly irritated red eyes and no history of trauma. She had flu-like symptoms 2 days ago.
343. A 36-year-old woman presents with red painful left eye, photophobia and decreased vision. Dendritic ulceration is noted on fluorescent stain.
344. A 7-year-old boy presents with painful left eye for 4 hours. Strong fluorescein uptake is noted in a well demarcated area of the cornea.

1. **False**
   Endogenous.

2. **True**

3. **False**
   Usually classified as endogenous, although an exogenous element is probable.

4. **False**
   Endogenous.

5. **False**
   Endogenous.

6. **True**

7. **True**

8. **True**

9. **False**
   The question asks for a good screening test and not an ideal screening test. If the positive and negative predictive values, the sensitivity and specificity all approach 100%, the test should be a diagnostic test rather than a screening test. A good screening test should have fairly high negative predictive value and sensitivity. However, the positive predictive value and the specificity (which depends not only on the test but also on the prevalence of the condition in that particular population) can be much lower if a good diagnostic test is available.

10. **False**

11. **True**
    One of the few absolute contraindications.

12. **False**
    Can try the transdermal route.

13. **False**

14. **False**
    Can try the transdermal route.

15. **False**
    The major reason for taking HRT is to protect the heart and bones.

16. **False**

17. **True**

18. **False**
    It is the experience of having thoughts put into one's mind by another person.

19. **False**
    It is the experience of hearing one's own thoughts being spoken out loud.

20. **True**

21. **False**
    About two-thirds. The rest have other characteristic symptoms such as catatonia or non-auditory hallucinations.

22. **True**

The acetabular roof is likely to be fractured unless the hip is held in adduction at the time of injury.

23. **True**

24. **False**

A passenger, whose knee or knees are struck by the dashboard when the car stops abruptly.

25. **False**

Short, adducted and internally rotated. The hip is most unstable in this posture.

26. **True**

Rare to start after 40 years of age; tumour should be suspected.

27. **True**

28. **False**

No diagnostic features.

29. **False**

It is no longer considered a *rubbish bin diagnosis* as the diagnosis can be made by meticulous history taking and careful physical examination.

30. **True**

For sedative and anti-cholinergic effects, *not* for antidepressant effect, as no antidepressant effect is documented for daily doses below 125–150 mg.

31. **True**

32. **False**

Normal or monocytosis.

33. **True**

34. **True**

35. **False**

Normal or basophilia.

36. **True**

37. **True**

38. **True**

39. **False**

The extent is increased.

40. **False**

Most think that the standard of care would be higher and the prescription rate would be lower.

41. **True**

42. **True**

43. **True**

44. **True**

Pseudocapsules are characteristic of fibroids.

45. False
Clean water at 38°C is acceptable.

46. False
No evidence of this.

47. True

48. True
Although this may be realised only after some of the debris is washed out.

49. True
Almost impossible to be sterile. A clean procedure is adequate.

50. False
Commonly.

51. True

52. True

53. False
Often palpable.

54. True

55. True

56. True

57. True
The Austin–Flint murmur.

58. False
Quincke's sign is capillary pulsation in nail beds.

59. True
Duroziez's sign, although uncommon.

60. True
Never mind what the Court Report recommendations are if you do not know. Just apply common sense to this type of historical question.

61. True

62. False
This is clearly not common sense.

63. True

64. True

65. True

66. True

67. True

68. False
MM is the normal phenotype. Individuals with ZZ have early onset chronic liver disease. Phenotypes of MS, SS or SZ or SZ are intermediate. Phenotype of null/null is associated with early onset emphysematous change.

69. **True**

70. **True**

71. **True**

72. **False**

73. **False**
Episodic vertigo.

74. **False**
Episodic vertigo.

75. **True**

76. **True**

77. **False**
Episodic vertigo.

78. **True**
If the diagnosis is confirmed and if the patient makes the informed decision to have no treatment.

79. **True**

80. **True**

81. **True**
The major adverse reaction is mucoid or mucopurulent vaginal discharge for up to 10 days postoperatively.

82. **True**

83. **True**
Salmonellosis is gastroenteritis caused by *Salmonella* species, as distinct from typhoid fever and paratyphoid fever (the enteric fevers).

84. **False**
Antibiotic is usually not indicated as the duration of *Salmonella* carriage might be prolonged. Cefuroxime or cefotaxime are used if the there is systemic disease, if the patient is immunocompromised, and for infants below the age of three months.

85. **True**
This is true for all types of gastroenteritis.

86. **True**

87. **False**
The Widal test is neither sensitive nor specific. Neutropenia is suggestive but not diagnostic. The yield of stool culture is high only during the second or third weeks. Blood culture is insensitive as the bacteraemia is episodic. Marrow culture remains the investigation giving the highest yield. The newest tools are monoclonal antibodies and PCR.

88. **True**

89. **False**
70%.

90. True

91. True

92. False
Women.

93. False
Every GP taking cervical smears should fully understand the terminology of cervical neoplasia, as such terms will appear in the cytology reports. CIN I, II and III correspond to mild, moderate and severe dysplasia respectively. These are histological diagnoses. The smear report gives a cytological diagnosis and a best guess for the histology only. CIS (stage 0 cervical carcinoma) is one step on from CIN III.

94. False
It is now believed that CIN and cervical carcinoma do not have any aetiological association with herpes. They are likely to be caused by HPV types 16, 18, 33 or 35.

95. False
Dysplasia is a histological term and diagnosis depends on tissue architecture and the morphology of individual cells. The corresponding cytological term is dyskaryosis. Thus the cervical smear may reveal moderate dyskaryosis and suggest moderate dysplasia, whereas the biopsy will confirm moderate dysplasia (CIN II).

96. False
It is best to reserve the term 'cancer' for at least CIS or other stages of cervical carcinoma. The sufferers can be informed that they have 'pre-cancers' of the cervix, which can progress to cancer.

97. False
All cases should be treated. Treatment may be postponed in pregnancy or in other exceptional circumstances.

98. True

99. False
Usually grow in pregnancy in response to high oestrogen levels.

100. False
Shrink at menopause because of low oestrogen levels.

101. False
Arise in the myometrium.

102. True

103. True

104. False
The upper third of the ulna is fractured.

105. False
Open reduction and internal immobilisation for adults. Surgery if closed reduction fails for children.

106. False
A fall on the hand.

107. False
The radial head is dislocated.

108. True
Though it is routinely performed.

109. False
Usually excised.

110. True

111. False
Not necessarily.

112. False
Usually employed.

113. True

114. True

115. True
Persistent infection with common or rare organisms.

116. False
Scanty.

117. True

118. True

119. False
After endocervical swab is taken. High vaginal swab is for diagnosis of vaginitis.

120. False
First, *T. vaginalis* is a protozoan and causes infestation rather than infection. Second, it causes strawberry ectocervicitis but very rarely causes infection above the ectocervix.

121. False
Outpatient management is appropriate for most cases. As many cases are sexually transmitted, contact tracing is important and may be more easily arranged by either the GP or the GUM clinic.

122. False
Caused by contact tracing being overlooked and thus reinfection.

123. True

124. True

125. True

126. True

127. False
About 40%.

128. True

129. True   169

130. True
The care component and the mobility component.

131. False
Is additional to most other benefits.

132. False
Was previously known as the attendance allowance and the mobility allowance.

133. True

134. True

135. True
Can be related or unrelated to food.

136. False
This is characteristic of a peptic ulcer. Vomiting does not relieve pain in functional dyspepsia.

137. False
Suggests duodenal ulcer or reflux oesophagitis.

138. False
Debatable, but unlikely to be true.

139. True

WHO (1985) diagnostic criteria for DM using 75 g oral glucose tolerance test.

Venous plasma (whole blood) glucose concentration mmol/L		
	Normal	Diabetic
Fasting	< 6.1 (5.6)	≥ 7.8 (6.7)
2 hours after glucose	< 8.9 (6.7)	≥ 11.1 (10.0)

140. True

141. False

142. False

143. False

144. False
The origin of the wrist extensors is affected.

145. False
When was the last time you saw this?

146. False
Lateral.

147. False
Repeated minor injuries.

148. False
Entrapment of a branch of the radial nerve.

149. False
No single definition for HT suits all purposes. The most important reason for defining HT is to provide a guide for subsequent treatment. Thus it can be defined as BP above a level which we have evidence (or reason to believe) that the benefits of treatment are more than the risks and disadvantages of treatment.

150. True
It is believed that the prevalence of complications increases with higher BP in a near-linear fashion. The same applies even to BPs below the common threshold (say 140/90) of treatment. The idea is that giving antihypertensive drugs to a person with a BP of 128/82 might still bring about some benefit. However, this is not done because if it were the disadvantages of treatment would outweigh the advantages of treatment.

151. False
Does not apply to malignant HT.

152. False
Not always, as the patient may have malignant HT in need of immediate drug treatment. For some patients with low initiatives, behavioural methods may not be most appropriate.

153. True

154. False
Ruptured or near-rupture.

155. True

156. True

157. False
Ruptured.

158. False
The other way round.

159. True

160. False
Behavioural therapy.

161. True
As in most psychiatric and psychological conditions.

162. True

163. True

164. False
Posterior.

165. False
Almost never.

166. False
Seen in the elderly.

167. True

168. True

171

169. **True**

170. **True**
Ringworm.

171. **True**
The first lesion in pityriasis rosea, although the trunk is more commonly involved. (However, pityriasis rosea is typical for its atypical presentations.)

172. **True**
Although the lower arm is more commonly involved.

173. **False**

174. **True**

175. **True**

176. **True**

177. **True**

178. **True**
Reducing the hepatic release of glucose and lowering insulin resistance.

179. **False**
Combination regimens are possible now.

180. **False**
Chlorpropamide is long acting among the first generation sulphonylureas.

181. **True**

182. **False**
Complete tear is commoner.

183. **True**

184. **False**
The commonest complication is lengthening of the tendon. Thus an equinus plaster is usually worn after approximation of the tendon ends.

185. **False**
Usually visible and palpable at 5 cm proximal to the insertion.

186. **False**

187. **True**

188. **True**

189. **True**
Many episodes may be related to the urethral syndrome.

190. **False**
It is recommended not to douche after intercourse, as douching might increase the risk of upper genital tract infections.

191. **False**
Shower may be better.

192. True

Individuals with HIV infection or AIDS can receive any vaccine, including live vaccines, other than BCG and yellow fever. Inactivated polio vaccine may be used instead of live oral polio vaccine.

193. False

194. False

195. True

196. False

197. False

198. True

Classic presentation.

199. False

200. False

201. False

202. True

Or as soon as they are able to comply, and reliable (i.e. repeatable) results are obtained.

203. False

The possibilities for this combination are:
- entirely normal hearing
- sensorineural hearing loss of similar severity on both sides
- very mild conductive hearing loss of similar severity on both sides.

204. True

205. False

All information obtainable from tuning fork tests can be obtained on the audiogram. The audiogram also differentiates hearing loss at different frequencies and gives quantitative assessment of the severity of hearing loss. However, the role of tuning fork tests as simple and quick screening tests cannot be replaced.

206. False

Tympanometry assesses middle ear and Eustachian tube function.

207. False

Alcohol.

208. True

209. False

DM is seen in only 15–20% of all patients.

210. True

211. True

212. True

213. **False**

214. **False**

215. **True**

216. **True**
Might be the most important factor.

217. **True**
As for other STDs.

218. **False**
Typical strawberry cervix.

219. **True**
True for male or female cases, true for adult or paediatric cases.

220. **False**
Oral metronidazole or nimovazole.

221. **True**

222. **False**
Colour is irrelevant.

223. **False**

224. **True**

225. **True**

226. **True**

227. **False**
Women are more prone.

228. **False**
This is a protective factor.

229. **False**
This is a protective factor.

230. **True**

231. **True**

232. **False**
Likely to be protective factors.

233. **False**
Screened by antibodies to Epstein–Barr virus capsid antigen, then confirmed by biopsy via fibreoptic nasopharyngoscope.

234. **False**
Epstein–Barr virus.

235. **False**
Little or late local symptoms.

236. **False**
Southeast China.

237. False
Radiotherapy is the mainstay of treatment for most cases.

238. False
Only hepatitis B specific immunoglobulin is available.

239. True

240. False

241. True
For immunocompromised children with contact history.

242. False
Although the use of respiratory syncytial virus specific immunoglobulin is being evaluated.

243. False

244. False
The benefit of preventing one case of rheumatic fever is likely to be balanced by one death caused by penicillin-induced anaphylaxis.

245. False
Most GPs still give antibiotics to children with otitis media. However, the outcome is generally unmodified. It may be worthwhile to identify at-risk groups who might benefit from antibiotics.

246. False
No advantage demonstrated.

247. False

248. True

249. True

250. False
4–6 weeks.

251. True

252. False
Highly infectious moist lesions in secondary syphilis.

253. True

254. True

255. False
Pox virus infection.

256. False
Drainage and marsupialisation.

257. False

258. True
Periorbital skin folds seen in chronic cases.

259. False

260. False

261. True
Rubbing the nose habitually in a superior fashion, seen in chronic cases.

262. True
Or a local authority residential home.

263. False
Applicable to danger through self-neglect or if endangering others.

264. True
Though in most cases a social worker applies to the director of public health.

265. True

266. False
No oral form exists as it is not absorbed.

267. True
The dose depends on renal function and the age and weight of the patient.

268. True

269. True

270. True

271. True
Like the apprehension test in recurrent dislocation of shoulder. If the patella is displaced laterally with the knee slowly flexed, resistance and apprehension of the patient are observed.

272. False
Weakness of the vastus medialis.

273. True

274. True

275. True

276. True

277. False
Sinus bradycardia.

278. True

279. False
Has been proved to have no value at all.

280. True

281. True

282. True
Phrenic nerve palsy.

283. True

284. True

285. **False**
Exploring such issues often leads to a fall in their prescription.

286. **False**

287. **True**
Holds for most patients.

288. **True**

289. **True**

290. **True**

291. **False**
Is a valid, reliable and convenient test of cure.

292. **False**
Both sensitivity and specificity are acceptable, in the region of 90–95%.

293. **True**
Serology cannot differentiate past inactive infection from active ongoing infection and cannot be employed as a test of cure.

294. **False**
Equipment necessary to collect the samples in the GP's surgery is simple; that needed to analyse the samples in the laboratory is sophisticated.

295. **False**
Usually too low, unless the insertion is avulsed.

296. **True**

297. **True**

298. **False**

299. **True**
Presents with jaundice and painful hepatomegaly.

300. **True**
Asymptomatic or subclinical, can be with hepatomegaly and chronic fatigue. The important fact concerning the GP is that it is reversible once alcohol is stopped.

301. **False**
The risk of hepatocellular carcinoma (HCC) is definitely increased in alcoholic cirrhosis, but HCC itself is not regarded as an alcoholic liver disease as the relationship is probably indirect.

302. **True**
One of the common causes of hepatitis, including fulminant hepatitis.

303. **True**

304. **True**

305. **False**
The Prader–Willi infant is hypotonic and feeding is difficult. There may be failure to thrive at that stage. At about 1 year of age he gradually turns hyperphagic and obesity then develops.

306. True

307. True
The three musculoskeletal complications of childhood and adolescent obesity.

308. False
Increased.

309. True

310. False
Absorption is adequate.

311. True

312. False
Pharmacokinetics is the delivery of the medication to the target organs. Oral HRT is pharmacologically inferior because of first-pass metabolism by the liver and thus less of the hormone reaches the target organs.

313. True

314. True

315. False

316. True

317. False
Suggests a mechanical problem.

318. True

319. False

320. False
Pathology in the atlas, axis or C3 vertebra.

321. True

322. False

323. True

324. False
Although their wishes are often respected.

325. True

326. H

327. A

328. A

329. B
Thus demonstrating the phenomenon of *anticipation*: the severity increases down the generations and age of onset of symptoms decreases down the generations.

330. D
Turner's syndrome.

331. H

332. C

333. F
Spontaneous. The role of genetic factors is uncertain.

334. C

335. C

336. D
The history of ankylosing spondylosis is a red herring.

337. B

338. K

339. D

340. A

341. F

342. L

343. H

344. C

MULTIPLE TRUE/FALSE QUESTIONS

Contraindications for HRT include

1. smoking
2. history of cervical cancer
3. history of ischaemic heart disease
4. history of thromboembolism
5. allergic contact dermatitis to the patches
6. history of breast cancer

Treatment of heart failure:

7. diuretics remain as the first line of drug treatment
8. vasodilators are contraindicated
9. angiotensin-converting enzyme inhibitors inhibit the conversion of angiotensin I to angiotensin II
10. lisinopril is characterised by a long half-life
11. inotropic agents have been shown to decrease mortality

Guidelines for sensible drinking.

12. half a pint of lager is 1 unit
13. the limit for women is 3–4 units a day
14. refraining on one day does not mean excess on another
15. a small glass of wine is 2 units
16. no more than 1–2 units once or twice a week is allowed for pregnant women

Common complaints in postcholecystectomy syndrome:

17. flatulence
18. right upper-quadrant pain
19. jaundice
20. intolerance of fatty foods
21. cholangitis

Gardnerella vaginal infection

22. may be associated with female homosexuality
23. may not need treatment
24. is associated with bacterial vaginitis
25. is an STD
26. typically causes glue cells in endocervical smear

Patients with dizziness

27. are mostly managed appropriately by their GPs
28. are frequently given an ENT diagnosis
29. are under-referred for specialist consultations
30. if referred, it is mostly to ENT specialists
31. are more likely to be referred if they consult their GP repeatedly

Antibiotic prophylaxis against endocarditis:

32. ampicillin is the usual drug of choice
33. oral antibiotic should be taken 4 hours before the procedure
34. probenicid should always be given
35. for patients with prosthetic valves, antibiotic is indicated for upper GI endoscopy
36. erythromycin or vancomycin can be used for patients allergic to penicillin

Vocal cord paralysis:

37. carcinoma of the bronchus may lead to right recurrent laryngeal nerve palsy
38. speech therapy may help
39. the cause is unidentifiable in most cases
40. recurrent laryngeal nerve palsy may be due to influenza
41. the abductor muscles are paralysed before the adductor muscles

Dupuytren's contracture

42. usually occurs in middle-aged men
43. is common in patients with DM
44. is inherited as an autosomal dominant disease
45. is related to alcoholic liver disease
46. nearly always affects both hands
47. begins with thickening of the palmar aponeurosis

Ovarian cysts:

48. corpus luteum cysts in tubal pregnancy usually occur on the same side
49. follicular cysts are usually neoplastic
50. luteinising hormone level is typically low in polycystic ovary syndrome
51. a theca luteal cyst is associated with a high HCG level

A 1-year-old child develops anaphylactic shock after MMR vaccination. Appropriate treatment includes

52. oral chlorpheniramine
53. intravenous adrenaline
54. nebulised bronchodilator
55. oral prednisolone
56. intramuscular hydrocortisone

The following causal associations are true:

57. adenovirus and sore throat
58. respiratory syncytial virus and bronchitis
59. parainfluenza virus and acute epiglottitis
60. rhinovirus and coryza
61. astrovirus and gastroenteritis

Peritonsillar abscess

62. is more common in children than adults
63. typically causes dysphagia
64. is safe to be drained by a GP
65. is an absolute indication for tonsillectomy
66. typically causes otalgia

Sleep apnoea syndrome:

67. marfanoid body proportion is a risk factor
68. early morning wakening is common
69. road traffic accidents are significantly increased
70. most sufferers can benefit from continuous positive airway pressure (CPAP)
71. thyrotoxicosis is a secondary cause

Screening tests performed in the UK:

72. Guthrie test for phenylketonuria
73. T_4 for congenital hypothyroidism
74. clinical examination for undescended testes
75. echocardiogram for congenital heart disease

Diphtheria:

76. the membrane is firm and adherent
77. the incubation period is 7–14 days
78. every diagnosed case should be admitted
79. neutropenia is characteristic
80. penicillin should be given to every diagnosed case

Recurrent epistaxis in an adolescent:

81. bleeding from the lateral nasal wall is more difficult to control
82. bleeding from Little's area is most likely
83. hereditary telangiectasia, an autosomal recessive disease, is a possible cause
84. no secondary cause is likely to be found
85. electrocautery may be performed under local anaesthesia

Symptoms of cervical ectropion:

86. mucoid vaginal discharge
87. low-back pain
88. deep dyspareunia
89. intermenstrual bleeding
90. mucopurulent vaginal discharge

The tetracyclines:

91. oxytetracycline is taken before meals as its absorption is reduced by chelation with calcium
92. it is advisable to prescribe tetracyclines with beta-lactams
93. they are effective against atypical chest pathogens like mycoplasma and chlamydia
94. local chlortetracycline commonly causes cutaneous sensitisation
95. renal impairment is not a contraindication

When the average consultation time is changed from 7.5 minutes to 10 minutes

96. the number of reconsultations might fall
97. the number of doctor consultations might fall
98. patient satisfaction might increase substantially
99. doctor satisfaction might increase substantially
100. the number of nurse consultations might fall

Differential diagnoses of ruptured ectopic pregnancy:

101. pelvic appendicitis
102. haemorrhage into an ovarian cyst
103. PID
104. haemorrhagic corpus luteum
105. torsion of an ovarian cyst
106. septic abortion

Infantile torticollis:

107. the face is tilted downwards on the unaffected side
108. deformity is usually apparent only when the child is three or four years old
109. the X-rays are likely to be normal
110. a history of low-segment caesarian section is common

Endometrial polyps

111. can be left without active treatment
112. are diagnosed by hysteroscopy
113. may be related to carcinoma of the ovary
114. are mostly shed at menstruation

After a myocardial infarction

115. low-dose aspirin has been shown to reduce the risks of further infarction and other vascular events
116. beta-blockers have been shown to reduce long-term mortality
117. angiotensin-converting enzyme inhibitors are contraindicated
118. empirical antiarrhythmic treatment is usually indicated
119. lipid-lowering agents have been shown to reduce the risk of further coronary events

Otosclerosis:

120. pregnancy makes it better
121. onset usually in fifth or sixth decades
122. most have a family history
123. the tympanic membranes usually appear sclerotic
124. paracusis is characteristic

Maintenance treatment in peptic ulcer should be considered in patients with

125. *Helicobacter pylori* infection
126. frequent symptomatic relapse
127. uncertain diagnosis
128. a history of life-threatening complications
129. a definite risk of future complications

Colorectal carcinoma:

130. a two-stage operation is usually the treatment of choice
131. surgery is contraindicated when hepatic secondary tumour(s) are present
132. family cancer syndromes are transmitted as autosomal dominant
133. regular checking of tumour markers is the screening method of choice for individuals with family cancer syndromes
134. stool for occult blood should be included in routine geriatric examinations

The Emergency Protection Order for children

135. legally gives the applicant parental rights
136. was known as Supervision Order in the past
137. can be applied for by the mother of the child
138. defines with whom the child is to live
139. places a child under the supervision of a local education authority
140. removes a child from a dangerous situation

Fractured calcaneum:

141. the ankle joint becomes immobile
142. examination must include the pelvis
143. the sufferer is usually a passenger in a car accident
144. a D-shaped bruise in the sole is characteristic

For the unmeasured DM diet, foods to be taken in moderation include

145. foods high in glucose and sucrose
146. meat extracts
147. fresh and dried fruit
148. tea and coffee
149. green vegetables

Management of mechanical low-back pain:

150. reassurance and simple analgesics are adequate for most sufferers
151. a firm mattress is usually recommended
152. transcutaneous nerve stimulation has been proved to be of benefit
153. chiropractic manipulation has been proved to be of benefit
154. tricyclic antidepressants are usually of no benefit

Acute otitis media in adults:

155. it can be a presenting sign of HIV infection
156. the maxillary sinus is a common source of infection
157. the absence of conductive hearing loss should cast doubt on the diagnosis
158. tenderness on pressing the mastoid antrum signifies mastoiditis
159. air flight is a precipitating factor

Helicobacter pylori

160. colonises the muscular layer of gastric antrum and body
161. is enteroinvasive
162. produces urease, converting ammonia to urea
163. has been proved to cause antral gastritis in children
164. infection is common in all communities

The following features occurring in naevi should initiate a referral:

165. bleeding
166. hairy naevus
167. ulceration
168. halo naevus
169. inflammation

Signs of acute eczema include

170. lichenification
171. exudation
172. scaling
173. pigmentation
174. fissuring

The GP contract includes the following as part of the terms and conditions of service of GPs:

175. undergraduate and postgraduate teaching
176. submission of an annual report
177. medical audits
178. the over-75s annual health checks
179. a plan for computerisation

Cervical carcinomas:

180. commonly cause an offensive watery discharge
181. cause early haematogenous spread
182. are mostly adenocarcinomas
183. commonly cause pain
184. commonly cause loss of weight

Signs of diabetic ketoacidosis include

185. bounding pulse
186. hypotension
187. sweating
188. air hunger
189. brisk reflexes

Management of psoriasis:

190. coal tar preparations are generally obsolete
191. calcipotriol stains skin and wallpaper
192. topical steroids cause tachyphylaxis and rebound and are generally contraindicated
193. dithranol is a vitamin D analogue
194. local retinoids are usually effective

Compartment syndromes (Volkmann's ischaemia):

195. all encircling splints and bandages should be removed immediately
196. surgical management is necessary in most cases
197. the extensor compartment of the forearm is most commonly affected
198. pain is often severe

Acute pancreatitis:

199. colicky pain is characteristic
200. onset of symptoms is usually sudden
201. perforated peptic ulcer and acute cholecystitis are important differential diagnoses
202. pancreatic pseudocyst is usually painful
203. pancreatic ascites is usually painful

Fibroids:

204. red degeneration is particularly common in pregnancy
205. most uterine fibroids descend during pregnancy
206. implantation of a fertilised ovum over a fibroid usually leads to ectopic pregnancy
207. fibroids may lead to premature onset of labour

A GP acting as a member of the school health service can expect to

208. provide health educational support to teachers
209. counsel children on individual or family health problems
210. assist in school sex education
211. deliver free posters and leaflets on health education

Cervical rib syndrome:

212. there may be wasting of small muscles of the hand
213. this is due to direct pressure on the vertebral artery and axillary nerve
214. this is present in every patient with cervical rib(s)
215. symptoms are common before the age of 20 years
216. it may be related to the Riley–Day syndrome

Common causes of conductive hearing loss in children:

217. barotrauma
218. chronic secretary otitis media
219. ear wax
220. congenital rubella syndrome
221. drug induced

Factors indicating a poor prognosis in proliferative glomerulonephritis:

222. nephritic-nephrotic syndrome
223. younger age
224. nephrotic syndrome
225. HT
226. poor renal function at presentation

The following would breach the General Medical Council guidelines on advertising by GPs:

227. informing the public that a GP has particular expertise in dermatology
228. writing to commercial organisations offering services as an occupational physician
229. having a regular advertisement in the local newspaper
230. placing copies of the practice information leaflet in public libraries
231. delivering the practice information leaflet to all residents in the practice area

Recommendations for an adult with frequent attacks of allergic rhinitis:

232. daily steroid nasal spray
233. vasoconstrictor nasal drops used when required
234. allergen avoidance
235. daily oral antihistamine
236. sodium cromoglycate nasal spray used when required

Laryngeal carcinoma:

237. most are subglottic
238. dysphagia is typically an early symptom
239. distant metastases are early and common
240. they are mostly adenocarcinomas
241. they are extremely rare in nonsmokers

Salpingitis:

242. the diagnosis is confirmed by endocervical swab for smear and culture
243. most cases present with acute low abdominal pain
244. most cases are febrile on presentation
245. a differential diagnosis is PID

The over-75s annual health check:

246. this should be an opportunity for health education and promotion
247. the task should be carried out by the GP himself
248. the frequency and amount of alcohol consumption should be assessed
249. a functional questionnaire is usually used

The following are notifiable infectious diseases:

250. meningitis
251. meningococcal septicaemia without meningitis
252. food poisoning
253. tuberculosis
254. HIV infection

Urinary symptoms in genital prolapse include

255. acute retention of urine
256. urge incontinence
257. urinary frequency
258. true incontinence
259. stress incontinence
260. incomplete emptying

Doctors who have completed their GP vocational training in the period 1990–95:

261. having children is the most important factor impeding career choice
262. virtually all are employed
263. availability of posts in the local area is a major factor impeding career choice
264. women are more likely than men to be working as principals
265. they take longer time to reach their final career destinations than previous cohorts

Recommended treatments for vulval viral warts:

266. cryotherapy
267. electrocautery
268. salicylic acid ointment
269. podophyllin resin
270. surgical excision

Educational changes in the 1990s are characterised by

271. the introduction of a national curriculum
272. segregation of children with complex special needs in special schools
273. schools working in partnership with parents
274. increased financial dependence of schools on the local authority

Antrochoanal polyps

275. arise in the maxillary antrum
276. may extend into the oral cavity
277. are usually multiple
278. can often be avulsed via the nasal route
279. manifest as an irregular swelling in the nasopharynx

Anterior dislocation of the shoulder:

280. the commonest nerve injury affects the circumflex nerve
281. X-ray is needed in every case
282. the arm is held adducted
283. the commonest cause is a fall on the hand
284. the contour of the shoulder appears rounded
285. the arm appears longer than the opposite side

Hepatitis A

286. does not have a chronic carrier state
287. cannot be spread by blood
288. causes higher mortality and more complications in pregnancy
289. is excreted in faeces for 2–3 weeks before the onset of symptoms
290. is best prevented by passive immunisation

Fracture-dislocation of the lower forearm:

291. a fall on the hand is the commonest cause
292. the lower end of the ulna is fractured
293. it is also known as Monteggia fracture-dislocation
294. the superior radioulnar joint dislocates
295. closed reduction is the treatment of choice for most cases

The 75 g oral glucose tolerance test:

296. a 4 hour fast is needed
297. the test cannot be applied to pregnant women
298. an unrestricted carbohydrate diet for at least 3 days before the test is
mandatory
299. the patient is allowed to perform normal walking activities during the test
300. the interpretation depends much on the renal threshold for glycosuria

Symptoms of PMS:

301. irritability
302. abdominal distension
303. migraine
304. asthmatic attack
305. swollen fingers and ankles
306. insomnia

Salivary gland tumours:

307. squamous cell carcinoma is the commonest malignant tumour
308. mucoepidermoid tumour is of intermediate malignancy
309. they should be considered malignant until proved otherwise
310. it is rarely possible to distinguish between benign and malignant tumours on
clinical grounds alone
311. adenolymphoma occurs almost exclusively in the submandibular gland

Causes of eosinophilia:

312. scabies
313. ulcerative colitis
314. tuberculosis
315. lymphoma
316. uncomplicated asthma

Anorexia nervosa:

317. the sufferer admits the problems but refuses any remedy
318. the weight loss is at least 25% of original body weight
319. the prevalence is higher in the upper social classes
320. many hate the process of preparing food
321. loss of interest in sex is a diagnostic criteria

Features of depression:

322. excessive feeling of guilt
323. sudden increased interests in hobbies
324. significant weight gain
325. unexpectedly increased libido
326. hypersomnia

GPs with more than 100 consultations per week

327. see more elderly patients
328. are generally more senior
329. see more patients with musculoskeletal problems
330. generally have more return consultations
331. see more patients with respiratory problems

Day centres for the elderly:

332. an attendance charge is usually levied
333. meals are usually provided
334. they are also known as day hospitals
335. their major function is rehabilitation for chronic diseases or after accidents

EXTENDED MATCHING QUESTIONS

Option list

(A) basal cell carcinoma
(B) chalazion
(C) dacryoadenitis
(D) dacryocystitis
(E) Kaposi's sarcoma
(F) malignant melanoma
(G) molluscum contagiosum
(H) squamous cell carcinoma
(I) stye
(J) viral wart
(K) xanthelesma
(L) xanthoma

Instruction

For each patient with an eye lesion, select the single most likely diagnosis. Each option can be used once, more than once, or not at all.

Items

336. A 25-year-old woman presents with painful reddish pimple on the lid margin.
337. A 35-year-old woman presents with warm painful swelling arising acutely in the superolateral aspect of the left upper eyelid.
338. A 56-year-old man presents with soft, yellowish skin lesions around both eyes.
339. A 45-year-old HIV-positive man presents with purplish nontender plaques around the eyes.
340. A 25-year-old man presents with a mildly tender, smooth, firm mass about 0.5 cm from the lower lid margin.
341. A 5-year-old boy has small nonpainful papules around the eyes. Umbilication is noted in some of the lesions.
342. An 11-year-old boy presents with warm painful swelling at the nasal aspect of the right lower eyelid.
343. A 59-year-old woman has a firm, pearly, ulcerated lesion on the right lower eyelid. A central dimple is evident.

Option list

(A) chicken pox
(B) drug rash
(C) guttate psoriasis
(D) HIV seroconversion illness
(E) measles
(F) papular urticaria
(G) pityriasis rosea
(H) pityriasis versicolor
(I) roseola infantum
(J) rubella
(K) scabies
(L) secondary syphilis

Instruction

For each patient with a rash, select the single most likely diagnosis. Each option can be used once, more than once, or not at all.

Items

344. A 10-year-old child has groups of itchy papules on the limbs for 2 weeks.
345. A 25-year-old woman has a generalised itchy rash after a tropical holiday. Patches of hyper- and hypopigmentation are seen.
346. A 26-year-old woman has five itchy papules on the trunk and face. She is afebrile. Examination reveals a vesicle on the hard palate.
347. A 9-month-old baby girl has macular facial rash on the fourth day of fever.
348. A 3-year-old child has maculopapular lesions on his chest on the fourth day of high fever. He is still febrile.
349. A 17-year-old young woman has non-itchy papules on the shoulder and upper trunk.
350. A 18-year-old man has generalised itch. Examination is unrewarding except for discovery of several papules on the penis.
351. An 18-year-old young man presents with a generalised mildly itchy rash with peripheral scaling. One single patch appeared 4 days before the generalised eruption.
352. A 19-year-old woman has fever, cervical lymphadenopathy, palatal petechiae and generalised macular rash.
353. A 19-year-old HIV-positive man has generalised macular rash and fever. Occipital lymph nodes are prominent.

1. **False**

2. **False**

3. **False**

4. **False**

5. **False**
   Other routes can be used.

6. **True**
   One of the few absolute contraindications.

7. **True**
   Generally true, except for heart failure caused by arrhythmias for which treatment of the arrhythmia is the first line of treatment.

8. **False**
   Nitrates reduce preload and hydralazine reduces afterload. However, their use is limited by tolerance and hypotension.

9. **True**

10. **True**

11. **False**
    They have been shown to increase mortality.

12. **True**

13. **False**
    2–3 units a day.

14. **True**

15. **False**
    1 unit.

16. **True**
    The threshold of fetal alcohol syndrome is very low.

17. **True**

18. **True**

19. **False**
    Uncommon.

20. **True**

21. **False**
    Uncommon.

22. **True**
    Unknown cause, but supported by epidemiology studies.

23. **True**
    Symptomatic cases should be treated. Treatment for asymptomatic cases, especially those in pregnancy, is highly controversial.

24. **False**

    Conventionally termed bacterial vaginosis because of the absence of inflammatory cells.

25. **False**

    May be associated with other STDs.

26. **False**

    Clue cells (epithelial cells surrounded by cocci), not glue cells. High vaginal smear, not endocervical smear.

27. **True**

28. **True**

29. **True**

    Especially elderly patients.

30. **True**

31. **True**

32. **False**

    Amoxycillin, for its broader coverage of Gram negatives.

33. **False**

    1 hour before.

34. **False**

35. **True**

36. **True**

37. **False**

    The course of the right recurrent laryngeal nerve is short and does not extend into the thorax.

38. **True**

    Particularly in cases of unilateral paralysis.

39. **False**

    Every effort must be made to identify the cause.

40. **True**

41. **True**

    Semon's law.

42. **True**

43. **False**

    Has a higher incidence only, but not common. Count how many of your DM patients have Dupuytren's contracture.

44. **True**

    For the familial cases.

45. **True**

46. **True**

47. True

48. True
Unless the fertilised ovum crossed over to the other side to be implanted, a rare event.

49. False
Not neoplastic, spontaneous disappearance.

50. False
The ratio of luteinising hormone to follicle-stimulating hormone is typically high, usually more than 3.0.

51. True

52. False
2.5 mg chlorpheniramine intramuscularly (preferable) or slow intravenously.

53. False
0.1 ml 1:1000 adrenaline intramuscularly (preferable) or subcutaneously. Intravenous route should be used only in extreme emergencies. Moreover, intravenous access is not easily available in the GP's surgery and valuable time will be lost.

54. True
If lower airway obstruction is present, although this is not the first priority.

55. False
Has much too slow an action in an emergency.

56. True
25 mg hydrocortisone intramuscularly (preferable) or slow intravenously.

57. True

58. False
Causes acute bronchiolitis in small children.

59. False
Most cases of croup are caused by parainfluenza virus. Acute epiglottitis is mostly caused by *Haemophilus influenza* type b, and has had a lower incidence since the introduction of universal Hib vaccination for infants and children in 1992.

60. True

61. True
Commonest after rotavirus.

62. False
Commoner in adults. Children below 4 years of age might have retropharyngeal abscess instead.

63. True

64. True

65. False
Debatable, but one episode is most likely not an indication.

66. **True**

67. **False**
Obesity is a risk factor.

68. **False**
The patient thinks that he has been asleep all night, but still feels
unrefreshed. Accompanying depression may lead to early morning wakening,
though.

69. **True**

70. **True**

71. **False**
Hypothyroidism.

72. **True**

73. **False**
Thyroid-stimulating hormone is used.

74. **True**

75. **False**
Clinical examination.

76. **True**

77. **False**
2–7 days.

78. **True**

79. **False**
Lymphocytosis.

80. **False**
Not if the patient is allergic. Erythromycin should be used instead.

81. **True**

82. **True**

83. **False**
It is an uncommon cause and is autosomal dominant.

84. **True**
Although no effort should be spared to exclude bleeding and clotting defects,
hypertension and local causes.

85. **True**

86. **True**

87. **True**

88. **True**
Although this is said to be possible with ectropion, another cause should be
actively looked for.

89. **True**

90. **True**
If the ectropion is secondarily infected.

91. **True**
True also for tetracycline and chlortetracycline.

92. **False**
Their effects are antagonistic. However, macrolides and beta-lactams may be prescribed concomitantly.

93. **True**
Although resistant strains are emerging.

94. **False**
Rarely.

95. **False**
All can exacerbate renal failure, except doxycycline and minocycline.

96. **True**

97. **True**

98. **False**
Likely to be marginally increased only.

99. **False**
Likely to be marginally increased only.

100. **False**
Rise.

101. **True**

102. **True**

103. **True**

104. **True**

105. **True**

106. **True**

107. **False**
On the affected side.

108. **True**

109. **True**

110. **False**
History of prolonged labour or breech delivery is common.

111. **False**
Removal, dilatation and curettage should be performed for histological confirmation of diagnosis.

112. **True**

113. **True**
Oestrogen-secreting tumours causing endometrial stimulation.

114. False

115. True

116. True

117. False
They might prevent onset of cardiac failure.

118. False
Specific agents should be given for specific arrhythmias.

119. True

120. False
Worse.

121. False
Second or third decades.

122. True

123. False
Usually normal.

124. True
Being able to hear better in noisy surroundings.

125. False
Inability to document or eradicate *H. pylori* infection is an indication to consider maintenance treatment.

126. True

127. False
No effort should be spared to ascertain the diagnosis.

128. True
Some physicians will consider a period of maintenance treatment.

129. True

130. False
Usually a one-stage procedure.

131. False
For symptomatic relief or in the hope of cure.

132. True

133. False
Regular colonoscopy.

134. False

135. False
The term 'parental right' is now replaced by 'parental responsibility'.

136. False
Was known as a Place of Safety Order.

137. **True**
Can be applied for by anyone. In most circumstances either a social worker or a worker of the National Society for the Protection of Cruelty to Children is involved.

138. **False**
This is then a Residence Order.

139. **False**
This is then an Education Supervision Order.

140. **True**

141. **False**
The ankle joint remains mobile. The subtalar joint is immobile.

142. **True**
There can be concomitant hip, pelvis or spine injuries.

143. **False**
Usually falls from a height landing on one or both heels.

144. **True**

145. **False**
Avoided altogether.

146. **False**
Eaten as desired.

147. **True**

148. **False**
Taken as desired.

149. **False**
Taken as desired.

150. **True**

151. **True**

152. **False**

153. **True**

154. **False**
Judicious use in chronic sufferers usually helps.

155. **True**
Almost anything can be.

156. **True**

157. **True**

158. **False**
Common in uncomplicated acute otitis media. Marked tenderness with other symptoms and signs suggests mastoiditis.

159. **True**
Barotrauma.

160. **False**
Epithelial mucous layer.

161. **False**

162. **False**
Urease converts urea to ammonia.

163. **True**

164. **True**

165. **True**

166. **False**
No need to refer if no change is noted.

167. **True**

168. **False**
Commonly seen, a normal phase in the life cycle of a naevus.

169. **True**
The other features are Asymmetry, irregular Border, irregular or change of Colour, increasing or large Diameter, and irregular or change of Elevation.

170. **False**
Sign of chronicity.

171. **True**

172. **True**

173. **False**
Sign of chronicity.

174. **False**
Sign of chronicity.

175. **False**

176. **True**

177. **True**

178. **True**

179. **False**

180. **True**

181. **False**
Early local or lymphatic spread.

182. **False**
Squamous cell carcinomas.

183. **False**
A late symptom.

184. **False**
Uncommon and late.

185. **False**
Weak pulse.

186. **True**

187. **False**
Suggestive of hypoglycaemia.

188. **True**
Hyperventilate to counteract the metabolic acidosis.

189. **False**
Diminished reflexes.

190. **False**
Acceptable to many patients.

191. **False**
Dithranol.

192. **True**
Except for face psoriasis, and combined with anti-candidial agents for flexural psoriasis.

193. **False**
Calcipotriol.

194. **False**
For acne only. Widespread psoriasis resistant to other treatments may respond to systemic retinoids given by a dermatologist.

195. **True**

196. **True**

197. **False**
Flexor compartment of the forearm.

198. **True**

199. **False**
Continuous.

200. **True**

201. **True**

202. **True**

203. **True**

204. **True**

205. **False**
Most uterine fibroids ascend during pregnancy and thus obstruction is a rare event.

206. **False**
Spontaneous abortion.

207. **True**

208. True

209. True

210. True

211. False
Responsibility of the Health Education/Promotion Unit.

212. True

213. False
Pressure on the subclavian artery and first thoracic nerve.

214. False
There must be at least some symptoms for this to be called a syndrome. The individual can be totally asymptomatic.

215. False
Rare before the age of 30 years.

216. False
Riley–Day syndrome is familial dysautonomia, a congenital dysfunction of the autonomic nervous system. It is totally unrelated to the cervical rib syndrome, although both can manifest with increased sweating. The autonomic dysfunctions in the cervical rib syndrome are caused by pressure effects on the first thoracic nerve and the sympathetic chain (Horner's syndrome).

217 True

218 True

219 True

220. False
Sensorineural.

221. False
Sensorineural.

222. True

223. False
Older age.

224. True

225. True

226. True

227. True

228. False

229. False

230. False

231. False

232. True
As prophylactic therapy.

233. False
Cause tolerance, rebound and tachyphylaxis, finally leading to rhinitis medicamentosa.

234. True

235. False
Causes tolerance. Should be used only in acute attacks.

236. True
Histamine-release inhibitor, should be used as prophylactic therapy as an alternative to steroid spray.

237. False
Most are glottic or supraglottic.

238. False
Late.

239. False
Uncommon.

240. False
Mostly squamous cell carcinomas.

241. True

242. False
Endocervical swab diagnoses endocervicitis and may suggest higher infections. The diagnosis of salpingitis is usually made on clinical grounds and is sometimes confirmed by laparoscopy.

243. False
The gynaecologists see only the tip of the iceberg. Actually most cases of salpingitis are subclinical and some are even asymptomatic.

244. False
See the answer to question 243.

245. False
PID is usually defined as salpingitis with or without endometritis resulting from an ascending infection and unrelated to surgery or childbirth. Thus, most cases of salpingitis are in fact PID.

246. True

247. False
Can be delegated to practice nurses.

248. True

249. True

250. True

251. True

   252. True

253. **True**

254. **False**

255. **True**

256. **True**

257. **True**

258. **False**
True continuous dribbling is usually the result of fistula formation.

259. **True**

260. **True**

261. **False**
Out-of-hours work.

262. **True**

263. **True**

264. **False**
Men are more likely.

265. **True**

266. **False**
Causes bullae formation, and may cause fistulae formation if warts extend into the vagina.

267. **True**

268. **False**
For cutaneous warts only, used for its keratolytic property.

269. **True**
Applied very meticulously to avoid irritant contact dermatitis.

270. **True**

271. **True**

272. **False**
Increased inclusion of such children in mainstream schools is advocated.

273. **True**

274. **False**
Increased financial independence.

275. **True**

276. **True**

277. **False**
Usually solitary.

278. **True**

279. **False**
Smooth regular swelling. Irregularity suggests carcinoma.

280. **True**

281. **True**
To confirm diagnosis, confirm reduction and exclude differential diagnoses such as fractures.

282. **False**
Abducted.

283. **True**

284. **False**
Angulated because of prominence of acromion.

285. **True**

286. **True**

287. **False**
Transient viraemia exists.

288. **True**

289. **True**
And up to 2 weeks afterwards.

290. **False**
Best prevented by active immunisation by vaccination if there is sufficient time.

291. **True**

292. **False**
The lower end of the radius is fractured.

293. **False**
Galeazzi. Monteggia is fracture-dislocation of the upper forearm.

294. **False**
The inferior radioulnar joint dislocates.

295. **False**
Open reduction and internal immobilisation.

296. **False**
Overnight fasting.

297. **False**
The diagnostic criteria are different.

298. **True**

299. **False**
Should remain seated and refrain from smoking.

300. **False**
Although glycosuria and ketonuria are routinely reported, only the whole blood or venous plasma sample results are used in the interpretation.

301. **True**
There are more than 60 symptoms listed.

302. **True**

303. **True**

304. **True**

305. **True**

306. **True**

307. **False**
Adenoid cystic carcinoma.

308. **True**

309. **True**

310. **True**

311. **False**
Almost exclusively in the parotid gland.

312. **True**

313. **False**
Causes normal CBC, or monocytosis or basophilia. Eosinophilia would suggest allergic colitis related to atopic conditions.

314. **False**
Causes monocytosis.

315. **True**

316. **True**

317. **False**
Typically denies the problems.

318. **True**
Or 25% below normal levels for age and height.

319. **True**

320. **False**
Many enjoy preparing food for others.

321. **True**
For male sufferers.

322. **True**

323. **False**
Loss of interest.

324. **True**
Or significant weight loss.

325. **False**
Decreased.

326. **True**
And also insomnia.

327. False
Insignificant difference.

328. True

329. False

330. True

331. False

332. True

333. True

334. False
Day centres are run by the local authority. Day hospitals are run by NHS Trusts.

335. False
The major role is to provide companionship.

336. I

337. C

338. K

339. E

340. B

341. G

342. D

343. A

344. F

345. H
The sunshine just darkens the normal skin and makes the rash apparent.

346. A
The papules will become vesicles within 12 hours.

347. E
The rash of measles typically starts on the face and gradually becomes generalised.

348. I
The rash will gradually spread to the abdomen, back and face. The fever will subside on the same day.

349. C
The lesions may not be scaly. A history of streptococcal sore throat is not always present. It is the symmetry with the typical distribution that counts.

350. K

351. G

352. B
Ampicillin-induced rash in infectious mononucleosis.

353. J
As he is already HIV-positive, he cannot have seroconversion illness again. Adult rubella is not that uncommon.

MULTIPLE TRUE/FALSE QUESTIONS

Problems related to a retroverted uterus:

1. menorrhagia
2. deep dyspareunia
3. low-back pain
4. dysmenorrhoea
5. recurrent spontaneous abortions
6. postmenopausal bleeding

Common causes of glomerulonephritis:

7. rheumatoid arthritis
8. DM
9. haemolytic-uraemic syndrome
10. Henoch–Schönlein purpura
11. cryoglobulinaemia

The following exceeds the ranges of sensible drinking:

12. three drinks of standard beer a day, male
13. two drinks of strong cider a day, female
14. one drink of brandy a day, male
15. one drink of super-strength lager a day, female
16. three drinks of brandy a day, male

Acute cholecystitis:

17. an obstructive cause is almost always present
18. plasma transaminases can be increased
19. Murphy's sign is right hypochondrial tenderness, worse on inspiration
20. leucocytosis is common
21. mortality in elderly patients may be as high as 10%

Definitions:

22. menopause is the physiological cessation of menstruation
23. primary amenorrhoea is amenorrhoea with a congenital or unidentified cause
24. primary fertility is the failure to attain pregnancy in the face of acceptable frequency of unprotected sex for a certain period and no previous history of pregnancy
25. secondary amenorrhoea is pathological amenorrhoea with a previous history of menses
26. primary infertility is infertility with unidentifiable cause
27. primary infertility is the failure to sustain a pregnancy in the face of acceptable frequency of unprotected sex for a certain period and no previous history of pregnancy

Differential diagnoses of cervical rib syndrome:

28. Poland's anomaly
29. carpal tunnel syndrome
30. Pancoast's tumour
31. ulnar tunnel syndrome
32. cervical spondylosis
33. Sprengel's anomaly

Colorectal carcinoma:

34. diet factors are relatively unimportant
35. it is the second commonest cancer of the GI tract in Western countries
36. obstructive symptoms are early in tumours of the ascending colon
37. pain is an uncommon symptom
38. mucus in stools and incomplete defaecation should alert the GP to the possibility of colorectal carcinoma at any age

Pathognomonic features of ectopic pregnancy are

39. dyspareunia
40. low abdominal pain
41. amenorrhoea
42. tender swelling on one side of uterus
43. shock
44. abnormal vaginal bleeding

Recurrent dislocation of the shoulder:

45. adolescents and young adults are particularly affected
46. diagnosis is by the apprehension test
47. it is caused by detachment of the glenoid labrum
48. it is prevented by prolonged immobilisation after anterior dislocation
49. the patient can often reduce the dislocation himself
50. conservative treatment is offered in most cases

Infectious mononucleosis:

51. the virus mainly affects T-cells
52. the atypical lymphocytes are T-cells
53. the incubation period is about 4–14 days
54. chronic fatigue is common after the infection
55. systemic steroid is contraindicated

Common causes of sensorineural hearing loss in adults:

56. barotrauma
57. presbycusis
58. otitis media
59. DM
60. acoustic neuroma

Cervical carcinoma:

61. the choice of treatment is mainly between surgery and chemotherapy
62. metastases beyond the pelvis signify stage 4 disease
63. stage 0 disease is CIN
64. cystoscopy is usually performed in every diagnosed case

Patients with psychogenic hyperventilation

65. have frequent sighing at rest
66. frequently present with the 'inability to take a deep breath'
67. typically have long breath-holding time
68. perform consistently well in spirometry studies
69. can present with carpopedal spasm caused by metabolic alkalosis

The following statements regarding adolescent health are true:

70. 80% of teenage pregnancies end in legal abortion
71. about 2–3% of secondary school children misuse drugs or solvents
72. about 50% of boys report a sexual experience before the age of 16 years
73. more adolescents now die from solvent abuse than from 'hard' drugs

For an unmeasured DM diet, foods to be eaten as desired include

74. tea and coffee
75. green vegetables
76. rolls and scones
77. fresh fruits
78. milk and cheese

The macrolide antibiotics:

79. erythromycin can be given by the parenteral route
80. erythromycin has a similar spectrum to penicillin
81. clarithromycin is usually given as a 3-day course for respiratory tract infections
82. azithromycin is usually given as a 3-day course for chlamydia genital tract infections
83. the serum half-life of azithromycin is long

Medical records:

84. computer records are acceptable as court evidence
85. keeping written medical records is a contractual but not a legal requirement
86. the Health Board usually reimburses 100% of the costs of computer hardware upgrades
87. medical records have to be kept for at least 5 years

Acute laryngitis:

88. may cause airway obstruction in small children
89. should be treated with antibiotics
90. is commoner in the winter months
91. is predisposed by alcohol
92. typically presents with drooling

Symptoms of hypoglycaemia include

93. confusion
94. headache
95. speech difficulty
96. weak pulse
97. dry skin and tongue

Ramsay Hunt syndrome

98. has a better prognosis for motor recovery than Bell's palsy
99. typically does not impair hearing
100. causes lower motor neuron lesion of the seventh cranial nerve
101. may affect the oculomotor nerve
102. is usually diagnosed by clinical features alone

The following symptoms suggest duodenal ulcer rather than gastric ulcer:

103. loss of weight
104. loss of appetite
105. nocturnal pain
106. pain exacerbated by food
107. pain exacerbated by hunger

Postgraduate education allowance:

108. distance learning courses may be eligible
109. the full allowance cannot be claimed by a part-time principal
110. sessions spent in minor surgery are eligible
111. courses leading to a diploma or a postgraduate degree are not counted

Vulval leucoplakia:

112. is not pre-malignant
113. manifests as thickening and atrophy of the vulval skin
114. is likely to recur after excision
115. is the female counterpart of balanitis xerotica obliterans in men
116. can extend to the perianal region

Carcinoma of the vulva

117. is related to HPV infection
118. commonly causes superficial dyspareunia
119. may be preceded by vulval intraepithelial neoplasia
120. spreads mainly by the lymphatic route
121. is usually treated by radial vulvectomy

All patients newly treated for HT should have

122. ECG
123. fasting cholesterol
124. liver function tests
125. renal function tests
126. Doppler studies for peripheral arterial diseases

Endometrial carcinomas

127. spread by direct invasion through the myometrium
128. are often anaplastic
129. are usually squamous cell carcinomas
130. usually spread haematogenously only in advanced cases
131. usually manifest with postmenopausal bleeding
132. are usually treated by chemotherapy

Colles' fracture:

133. the distal part of the radius is usually displaced in a pronated fashion
134. it causes 'dinner-fork' deformity because the distal part of the radius is dislocated posteriorly
135. open reduction is the treatment of choice for most patients
136. it is also known as backward Monteggia
137. the distal part of the radius is usually in ulnar deviation
138. carpal tunnel syndrome is rare

Common causes of ascites in adults:

139. hepatic tumours
140. protein-losing enteropathy
141. cardiac failure
142. cirrhosis of liver
143. hypothyroidism

Chronic otitis media:

144. cholesteatoma forms within the inner ear
145. mucoid discharge signifies tympanic membrane perforation
146. complications are common in tubotympanic disease
147. central perforation is typical in tubotympanic disease
148. the success rate of myringoplasty is high

Substance abuse:

149. LSD is the most commonly used hallucinogen
150. some individuals are better maintained on regular oral methadone than gradual withdrawal
151. glue sniffing rarely leads to regular use or dependence
152. LSD use rarely leads to chronic psychosis
153. ecstasy is rarely addictive

Androgenetic alopecia:

154. no effective treatment is available for most sufferers
155. bitemporal recession is typical
156. may occur in two phases
157. systemic minoxidil is licensed for its treatment
158. crown involvement is typical

The stillbirth rate

159. together with the rate of babies dying in the first 12 months of life is the infant mortality rate
160. is the number of babies born dead with a gestational age of at least 28 weeks per 1000 total births
161. together with the neonatal mortality rate is the perinatal mortality rate
162. is the number of babies born dead with a gestational age of at least 24 weeks per 1000 live births
163. together with the rate of babies dying in the first 28 days of life is the perinatal mortality rate
164. is affected mostly by the standard of antenatal care

HRT:

165. no beneficial effect on the bones has been proved by taking HRT for 2–3 years
166. giving progestogen decreases the beneficial effects on the CVS exerted by the oestrogen
167. long-term use of HRT can reduce the incidence of coronary heart diseases by as much as 40%
168. to give HRT to relieve menopausal symptoms only, the lowest effective dose of oestrogen should be given for the shortest effective period

Risk factors for acute pancreatitis:

169. gallstones
170. alcohol
171. hypocalcaemia
172. hyperlipoproteinaemia
173. mumps

Overuse syndromes:

174. 'shin splints' may be caused by tendinitis
175. Achilles tendinitis in a young male athlete suggests seronegative arthropathy
176. dancers and runners often complain of pain around the greater trochanter of the femur
177. 'jumper's knee' mainly affects the posterior knee bursas

Common factors causing flare-ups of psoriasis include

178. food
179. infection
180. sunlight
181. emotion
182. trauma

Uterine fibroids:

183. fibroids usually shrink after menopause
184. myomectomy may impair fertility
185. vaginal hysterectomy should be considered if the uterus is grossly enlarged with multiple fibroids
186. menorrhagia progressively getting worse is the common indication for surgery

A diagnosis of DM is made by

187. two incidents of glycosuria and ketonuria
188. a random blood glucose of 16.9 mmol/L
189. HbA$_1$ of 13.0%
190. fasting blood glucose of 6.5 mmol/L
191. HbA$_1$ of 8.5%

The over-75s annual health check should include assessment of

192. mobility
193. mental function
194. sensory function
195. social circumstances
196. use of medications
197. physical condition

Simple Doppler ultrasonography for peripheral arteries

198. should always be performed before applying compression to the lower limbs
199. is easily available in GP surgeries
200. is the first investigation of choice in peripheral arterial disease
201. is usually adequate to be performed on one artery on each limb
202. guides treatment in chronic leg ulcers

Tinnitus:

203. if due to otosclerosis may not be relieved by stapedectomy
204. may be audible to the GP
205. it is usually aggravated by fatigue
206. it is pulsating in glomus jugulare tumour
207. if caused by ototoxicity, it is usually permanent

Low-back pain:

208. acute onset signifies a systemic or medical cause
209. most resolve in 1–2 weeks
210. depression is a recognised risk factor
211. chronic pain of more than 3 months accounts for about one-third of all cases
212. early mobilisation is recommended for most patients

Frequent attenders

213. frequently present with psychosomatic complaints
214. are more likely to have marital problems
215. rarely have genuine physical and psychosocial needs
216. frequently cause a dysfunctional doctor–patient relationship
217. are more likely to have stressful life events

Wrist ganglia:

218. they are solid firm lesions
219. they are usually painful
220. they usually arise from synovial herniation from a joint
221. the anterior wrist is most commonly affected

Features suggesting life-threatening asthma:

222. pulsus paradoxicus
223. use of accessory muscles
224. peripheral cyanosis
225. peak flow rate less than 50% of best or predicted value
226. change of conscious level

Target groups for hepatitis A vaccination include

227. travellers to Australia
228. contact cases of hepatitis A
229. homosexuals
230. babies born to mothers with HAV IgG +ve
231. babies born to mothers with HBeAg +ve

Benign positional vertigo

232. typically causes vertigo of short duration
233. may be related to head injury
234. is believed to be a degenerative disease
235. is usually accompanied by nystagmus
236. may be related to cerebellar tumour

For immunisations:

237. two live vaccines should either be given on the same day or at least 3 weeks apart
238. two inactivated vaccines should either be given on the same day or at least 1 month apart
239. live vaccines should be given 3 months before or 3 weeks after immunoglobulins
240. live vaccines are generally contraindicated for individuals with HIV infection
241. systemic antibiotic treatment is a contraindication to live vaccines

Meal-on-wheels service:

242. elderly people attend the club in wheelchairs
243. meals are usually provided only 2–3 times per week
244. preparation, delivery and storage are practical problems
245. some delay is inevitable

Common clinical features of infective endocarditis include

246. Roth's spots
247. cardiac failure
248. Osler's nodes
249. subconjunctival haemorrhage
250. haematuria

Elderly people with atrial fibrillation:

251. most would prefer blood testing for anticoagulation in a hospital
252. they have more disability than the general elderly population
253. compliance in taking anticoagulants is a major difficulty
254. most would accept anticoagulation treatment to prevent cerebrovascular events
255. cognitive impairment is not different from the general elderly population

Cervical spondylosis:

256. neurological signs in the lower limbs cast doubt on the diagnosis
257. the pain is worse in the evening and at night
258. lipping is caused by hypertrophy of the disc cartilage
259. changes in X-rays are seen in most patients

Nasal polyps

260. are common in children
261. are usually bilateral
262. can be removed under local anaesthesia
263. rarely cause nasal obstruction
264. rarely disappear on nasal steroid spray

Characteristic signs of a right temporal lobe abscess:

265. visual hallucinations
266. right upper-quadrant homonymous hemianopia
267. dysphasia
268. dysdiadochokinesis
269. right side of the face and arm paralysis

Angina

270. may radiate to the lower arms
271. usually interrupts breathing and coughing
272. usually relieves on bending the trunk
273. is usually very sudden in onset
274. accompanied by breathlessness suggests myocardial infarction

Regarding adoption:

275. honesty with adopted children is advocated
276. adoption while retaining contact with birth relatives should be discouraged
277. open adoption with the birth parent actively involved in selecting and meeting adopters is increasingly practised in some Western countries
278. adopters usually receive an allowance from the adoption agency

The basal body temperature chart:

279. a rise of 0.4–0.5°C is seen about 12 hours after ovulation
280. the temperature should be taken first thing in the morning before the woman leaves her bed
281. the chart is an indirect indication of oestrogen sufficiency in the second half of the menstrual cycle
282. electronic thermometers are less accurate than mercury thermometers and should not be used

Risk factors for carcinoma of the cervix:

283. multiple sexual partners
284. late first sexual intercourse
285. partner with HPV infection of the skin
286. Caucasians
287. history of vulval viral warts

Consultations for cough

288. are commoner in the unemployed
289. are commoner in men
290. are associated with greater anxiety and stressful events
291. are commoner in children
292. are commoner in manual groups

Symptoms of ovarian tumours:

293. low-back pain
294. palpable ovarian cyst
295. low abdominal pain
296. central dullness on percussion
297. menstrual irregularity
298. abdominal distension

Abuse of elderly people:

299. theft of money or property is regarded as a form of abuse
300. the over 75s annual health check should be used to explore possible abuse
301. the prevalence is about 20%
302. the GP has a central role in its prevention and treatment
303. neglect of basic needs is a type of abuse

Acute maxillary sinusitis:

304. antral washout should not be performed in the acute phase
305. it is one of the complications of whooping cough
306. ampicillin is the antibiotic of choice for most cases
307. metronidazole may be needed in some cases
308. cheek swelling and tenderness over the antrum are characteristic

Descriptions of skin lesions:

309. a macule is a small flat area of unaltered colour or texture
310. a bulla is a circumscribed elevation of skin over 0.5 cm in diameter and containing fluid
311. a papule is a solid mass in the skin larger than 0.5 cm in diameter
312. a pustule is a localised collection of pus in a cavity, more than 1 cm in diameter
313. a purpura is a pinhead-sized macule of blood in the skin

Cervical ectropion:

314. columnar epithelium is replaced with squamous epithelium
315. it is a common cause of postcoital bleeding
316. there is a relative lack of mucus-secreting glands
317. an important differential diagnosis is simple cervical erosion
318. the external cervical os is mainly affected

Factors in reflux oesophagitis include

319. obesity
320. cigarette smoking
321. history of cardiomyotomy
322. pregnancy
323. alcohol

Practices implementing recommended evidence-based changes in prescribing

324. are more likely to use clinical protocols
325. are more likely to be fundholding
326. have GPs with more innovative approaches
327. are more likely to have disease registers
328. are more likely to use computers

The following associations are true in entrapment neuropathy:

329. radial nerve palsy and sensory loss of posterior aspect of upper arm and forearm
330. carpal tunnel syndrome and sensory loss in the little finger
331. peroneal nerve compression and weakness of plantarflexion of foot
332. ulnar nerve compression at elbow and weakness of small muscles of the hand
333. radial nerve palsy and weakness of pronator teres

Parkinson's disease:

334. greasy skin is characteristic
335. the tremor is of about 4.6 Hz
336. clasp-knife rigidity is characteristic
337. the tremor is worse on voluntary movements
338. clinical features can be unilateral initially

EXTENDED MATCHING QUESTIONS

Option list

(A) angina
(B) dissecting aneurysm
(C) drug related
(D) gastro-oesophageal reflux
(E) malingering
(F) Munchausen's syndrome
(G) musculoskeletal pain
(H) myocardial infarction
(I) pericarditis
(J) pleuritic pain
(K) pneumothorax
(L) psychosomatic

Instruction

For each patient with chest pain, select the single most likely diagnosis. Each option can be used once, more than once, or not at all.

Items

339. A 28-year-old man complains of left-sided chest pain and shortness of breath for 1 day. The onset was sudden. Examination reveals normal chest findings with no hyper-resonance.

340. A 78-year-old woman complains of chest pain and breathlessness not relieved by nitrates. Examination reveals sinus bradycardia.

341. A 28-year-old man has a cough and purulent sputum. He complains of localised left posterior chest pain related to sleeping posture.

342. A 35-year-old woman presents with a cough and left-sided chest pain aggravated by coughing. Examination reveals diffuse crepitation, no rhonchi and no pleural rub.

343. A 38-year-old man complains of central chest pain relieved by nitrates prescribed for his father's angina. The pain is worse after hot foods and is precipitated by exercise.

344. A 68-year-old man with HT and DM complains of choking and breathlessness on exertion, remitting at rest. The sensation is worse after large meals. Resting ECG is normal.

345. A 35-year-old woman complains of a 'tearing' pain in the back. She was diagnosed as having atrial septal defect secundum by a cardiologist. ECG strip brought by her reveals right bundle branch block and right axis deviation. Examination reveals normal heart sounds and no murmur.

Option list

(A)   fourth cranial nerve palsy
(B)   intermittent non-paralytic squint
(C)   latent squint
(D)   left convergent non-paralytic squint
(E)   left divergent non-paralytic squint
(F)   myasthenia gravis
(G)   normal (no squint, no pseudosquint)
(H)   pseudosquint
(I)   right convergent non-paralytic squint
(J)   right divergent non-paralytic squint
(K)   sixth cranial nerve palsy
(L)   third cranial nerve palsy

Instruction

For each patient with a squint, select the single most likely diagnosis. Each option can be used once, more than once, or not at all.

Items

346. A 3-year-old boy presents with apparently deviating eyes and epicanthic folds. His left eye deviates laterally when his right eye is covered.

347. A 45-year-old woman has double vision. She has right ptosis and her right eye looks down and out.

348. A 6-year-old boy has apparently deviating eyes. He has double vision. He has no ptosis. Pupils are equal in size.

349. A 6-year-old boy has apparently deviating eyes. There is no abnormal eye movement on the cover test. The visual acuities are normal.

350. A 3-year-old girl has a manifest squint. Her right eye deviates medially when her left eye is covered.

351. A 23-year-old girl has poorly managed chronic otitis media with cholesteatoma. She develops double vision.

352. A 2-year-old boy has a manifest squint. His left eye deviates laterally when his right eye is covered. His right eye does not move when his left eye is covered.

353. A 4-year-old boy is noticed by his mother to have a squint whenever he is tired. Cover and uncover tests when he is alert reveals no abnormal eye movement.

354. A 7-year-old girl does not exhibit abnormal eye movement in the cover test. Her left eye deviates from a lateral to the central position on being uncovered.

1. **True**

2. **True**

3. **True**

4. **False**
    The incidence is not increased.

5. **True**

6. **False**
    Not related.

7. **False**
    Uncommon.

8. **True**

9. **False**
    Rare.

10. **True**

11. **False**
    Rare.

12. **True**
    Total of 6 units, exceeding the limit of 3–4 units/day for men.

13. **True**
    Total of 4.7 units, exceeding the limit of 2–3 units/day for women.

14. **False**
    Total of 1 unit.

15. **True**
    Total of 4 units.

16. **False**
    Total of 3 units.

17. **False**
    10% have no obstruction and the cause is unclear.

18. **True**

19. **True**

20. **True**

21. **True**

22. **False**
    Menopause is the presumed permanent cessation of menstruation. It can be physiological, pathological, drug-induced or surgical.

23. **False**
    It is the absence of menstruation at a certain age (usually 17 years) with no previous history of menses at all.

24. **False**
    Read carefully. The statement is a correct definition for primary infertiliy, not primary fertility.

25. **False**
    Usually defined as no menses for 6 (some say 12) months with a previous history of menses. Secondary amenorrhoea needs not be pathological; it includes physiological causes such as pregnancy.

26. **False**
    It is infertility with no previous history of pregnancy.

27. **False**
    It is the failure to attain, not sustain, a pregnancy, and therefore does not include recurrent spontaneous abortions.

28. **False**
    Although there may be radial nerve aplasia in Poland's anomaly, the symptoms and signs are almost totally different.

29. **True**

30. **True**

31. **True**

32. **True**

33. **False**
    Incompletely descended scapula(e). The presentation is completely different to that of cervical rib syndrome.

34. **False**

35. **False**
    The commonest.

36. **False**
    Descending and sigmoid colon.

37. **False**
    Common, present in 60–70% of all patients at some time.

38. **False**
    True only for patients above the age of 40 years or those with familial history of tumour syndromes. Below 30–35 years of age, these two symptoms are highly suggestive of IBS, and in fact are two of the six Manning's criteria for IBS. The other criteria are: recurrent abdominal pain relieved by defaecation, frequent defaecation, abdominal distension and audible borborygmi. An interesting fact here is the difference in terminology for the same symptoms at different ages. Below the age of 30–35 years, it is known as incomplete defaecation; after 40 years of age it should be documented as tenesmus.

39. **False**
    Pathognomonic means that the clinical feature occurs only in a particular condition. It virtually never occurs in other conditions. A pathognomonic feature can be common or uncommon in that condition. The features listed are all possible in ectopic pregnancy. Tender swelling on one side of the uterus is highly suggestive of ectopic pregnancy but can occur in other conditions such as torsion of an ovarian cyst.

40. **False**

41. **False**

42. **False**

43. **False**

44. **False**

45. **True**

46. **True**
The shoulder is passively and laterally rotated while held in abduction. Immediate resistance is felt.

47. **True**

48. **False**

49. **True**

50. **False**
Active surgical management to strengthen the shoulder joint is needed.

51. **False**
B-cells.

52. **True**
Despite the fact that mainly B-cells are infected, the atypical cells are T-cells.

53. **True**

54. **True**
But full blown myalgic encephalomyelitis (ME) is less common.

55. **False**
Severe tonsillar enlargement causing dysphagia or breathing difficulty necessitates admission for intravenous corticosteroids.

56. **False**
Conductive hearing loss.

57. **True**

58. **False**
Conductive hearing loss.

59. **False**
An uncommon cause of sensorineural hearing loss.

60. **False**
An entity seen in neurofibromatosis type 2. Causes sensorineural hearing loss but is uncommon.

61. **False**
Surgery and radiotherapy.

62. **True**

63. **False**
Stage 0 is CIS.

64. **True**
To assess for spread to the urinary bladder.

65. **True**

66. **True**

67. **False**
Breath-holding time is usually short.

68. **False**
Results are inconsistent.

69. **False**
Respiratory alkalosis.

70. **False**
Only one-third end in legal abortion.

71. **False**
About 16%.

72. **True**

73. **True**

74. **True**

75. **True**

76. **False**
To be taken in moderation.

77. **False**
To be taken in moderation.

78. **False**
To be taken in moderation.

79. **True**
Intravenous form is available.

80. **True**
It thus can be used in place of penicillin in penicillin-allergic individuals.

81. **False**
Usually given as 7–10 day courses.

82. **False**
Usually given as 1-dose course of 1 g, effective against *Chlamydia trachomatis* serovars D–K (non-gonococcal urethritis and mucopurulent cervicitis) and *Neisseria gonorrhoeae*.

83. **True**
And therefore given twice daily for 3 days for respiratory tract infections.

84. **True**

85. **False**

86. **False**

87. **True**

88. **True**

89. **False**
Usually viral in origin.

90. **True**

91. **True**

92. **False**
Suggests acute epiglottitis.

93. **True**

94. **True**

95. **True**

96. **False**
Full bounding pulse.

97. **False**
Moist skin and tongue.

98. **False**
Worse.

99. **False**
Hearing impaired.

100. **True**

101. **False**
Cranial nerve VII is the most often affected. Rarely cranial nerves V, VI, IX, X and XII may also be affected.

102. **True**

103. **False**
Suggests gastric ulcer or gastric carcinoma.

104. **False**
Suggests gastric ulcer.

105. **True**

106. **False**
Suggests gastric ulcer.

107. **True**

108. **True**

109. **False**

110. **False**

111. **False**

112. **False**
Is pre-malignant.

113. **False**
Thickening and hypertrophy of the vulval skin.

114. **True**

115. **False**
Lichen sclerosis et atrophius is the female counterpart of balanitis xerotica obliterans.

116. **True**

117. **True**

118. **False**
Often subclinical or asymptomatic for long periods.

119. **True**
Vulval intraepithelial neoplasia (VIN) precedes carcinoma of the vulva like vaginal intraepithelial neoplasia (VAIN) precedes vaginal carcinoma and CIN precedes cervical carcinomas.

120. **True**

121. **True**

122. **True**
For ischaemic changes and signs of ventricular hypertrophies.

123. **True**

124. **False**

125. **True**

126. **False**
Only if history or physical findings suggest peripheral arterial disease.

127. **True**

128. **False**
Often well differentiated.

129. **False**
Adenocarcinomas.

130. **True**

131. **True**

132. **False**
Surgery.

133. **False**
In a supinated fashion if there is any rotational displacement.

134. **True**

135. **False**
Closed reduction under anaesthesia for most patients.

136. **False**
Colles' fracture is transverse fracture of the radius less than 2.5 cm from the wrist. Backward Monteggia, like Monteggia, is fracture-dislocation involving the upper third of the forearm. The radial head and the distal part of the ulnar are displaced backwards in backward Monteggia.

137. False
The deviation is lateral (radial) if any is present.

138. True
Carpal tunnel syndrome is a recognised but rare complication of Colles' fracture.

139. True

140. False
Uncommon.

141. True

142. True

143. False
Rare.

144. False
Middle ear.

145. True

146. False
Uncommon.

147. True

148. True

149. True

150. True

151. True

152. True

153. True

154. True
The GP's job is to turn 'sufferers' into non-sufferers by helping them to accept their hair loss as a normal process of life.

155. True

156. True
An early phase that occurs when people are aged in their late 20s is common, though not commonly realised.

157. False
A minority responds temporarily to topical minoxidil.

158. True

159. False
The infant mortality rate is the number of infants dying in the first 12 months of life per 1000 live births.

160. False
At least 24 weeks.

161. **False**
     The neonatal mortality rate is the number of infants dying in the first 28 days of life per 1000 live births.

162. **False**
     Per 1000 total births.

163. **False**
     The perinatal mortality rate is the stillbirth rate and number of babies dying in the first 7 days of life.

164. **True**

165. **True**
     It takes at least 5–10 years before any beneficial effect is demonstrable.

166. **True**
     However, the overall effect is still protective for the CVS.

167. **True**

168. **True**
     Unlike for the prevention of osteoporosis and cardiovascular diseases. Thus the reason for starting HRT must be clear to both the patient and the GP.

169. **True**

170. **True**

171. **False**
     Hypercalcaemia.

172. **True**

173. **True**

174. **True**
     Manifests with pain in the lower medial aspect of the tibia.

175. **False**
     Although Achilles tendinitis may occur in ankylosing spondylitis in young men, it is most likely caused by overstress in a young athlete.

176. **True**
     'Trochanteric bursitis'.

177. **False**
     Affects the patellar ligament.

178. **False**
     Rarely related to food.

179. **True**
     Streptococcal infection followed by guttate psoriasis.

180. **False**
     Uncommon. 90% improve in response to sunlight; 10% worsen in response to sunlight.

181. **True**

182. **True**
     Köbner phenomenon.

183. **True**

184. **True**
     Usually because of adhesions.

185. **False**
     Abdominal hysterectomy should be considered in this case, if the woman is over 40 years of age and has completed her family.

186. **True**

187. **False**
     75 g oral glucose tolerance test (OGTT) is indicated.

188. **True**
     Above 14.0 mmol/L is diagnostic, although the HbA_1 can be checked concomitantly.

189. **True**
     Above 9.0% is diagnostic, although random blood glucose can be checked concomitantly.

190. **False**
     OGTT is indicated if fasting glucose is between 6.0 and 8.0 mmol/L.

191. **False**
     OGTT is indicated if HbA_1 is between 8.0 and 9.0%.

192. **True**
     These six aspects cover almost everything and it is difficult to quote an example that is not included in the assessment.

193. **True**

194. **True**

195. **True**

196. **True**

197. **True**

198. **True**

199. **True**
     It is relatively inexpensive. Without it, treatment of any chronic leg ulcer may be difficult as it is then impossible to exclude peripheral arterial disease. Applying compression therapy to a leg ulcer caused by venous insufficiency is beneficial, but applying this in arterial disease causes further ischaemia and gangrene. It is difficult to exclude arterial insufficiency by physical examination alone.

200. **True**

201. **True**
     Usually both brachial and both dorsalis pedis arteries, although the posterior tibial is sometimes used.

202. True

203. True

204. True
If caused by an aneurysm.

205. True

206. True

207. True

208. False
Signifies a mechanical cause. Those of medical or systemic causes are usually insidious in onset.

209. True

210. True
Likely to be a predisposing, precipitating and a perpetuating factor.

211. False
Less than 5%.

212. True

213. True

214. True

215. False
Usually.

216. True

217. True

218. False
Cystic and commonly transilluminate.

219. False
Pain is minimal or absent.

220. False
Usually from small bursas in the joint capsule or fibrous tendon sheath.

221. False
The back of the wrist.

222. False
Proved to have no relevance to the severity of the attack.

223. False
Suggests severe asthma only.

224. False
Central cyanosis.

225. False
Suggests severe asthma. Peak flow rate of less than 33% of best or predicted value suggests life-threatening asthma.

226. **True**

227. **False**
Travellers to countries outside northern and western Europe, North America, Australia and New Zealand.

228. **True**

229. **True**
Any oral–anal contact causes a risk.

230. **False**
The mother is immune to hepatitis A.

231. **False**
Hepatitis B vaccination and hepatitis B immunoglobulin should be given.

232. **True**
Transient when the head is turned.

233. **True**
Some cases follow head injury.

234. **True**

235. **True**

236. **False**

237. **True**
To two different sites if given on the same day.

238. **False**
Generally no interaction exists between inactivated vaccines.

239. **False**
3 weeks before or 3 months after immunoglobulins.

240. **False**
Even individuals with AIDS can be given most vaccines except BCG and yellow fever. The inactivated injected form of polio vaccine is commonly used, although the oral live form is not absolutely contraindicated.

241. **False**
It is one of the many false contraindications, others being prematurity, low birth weight, atopic diseases, steroid inhalation treatment and uncomplicated afebrile upper respiratory tract infections.

242. **False**
Meals are brought to their homes on wheels.

243. **True**

244. **True**

245. **True**

246. **False**
Uncommon.

247. **True**

248. **False**
Uncommon.

249. **False**
Uncommon.

250. **True**

251. **False**
Outside the hospital.

252. **False**
No significant difference.

253. **False**
Can be overcome.

254. **True**

255. **True**

256. **False**
The lower limbs may display signs of upper motor neuron lesion.

257. **False**
Worse in the early morning.

258. **False**
Lipping occurs in the bones. It is caused by hypertrophy of the vertebral bodies.

259. **True**
But the reverse is not true: most people with such X-ray changes have no symptoms. The extent of X-ray changes usually bears no direct relationship to the severity of the symptoms.

260. **False**
Rare.

261. **True**

262. **True**

263. **False**
Commonly.

264. **True**
They just shrink.

265. **False**
A sign of occipital lobe lesions. Temporal lobe lesions cause hallucinations of taste and smell.

266. **False**
Left upper-quadrant homonymous hemianopia.

267. **False**
Common for left-sided lesion.

268. **False**
An inability to perform two coordinating movements simultaneously. Seen in cerebellar lesions.

269. False
Left side of the face and arm paralysis.

270. True

271. False
This describes pleuritic pain.

272. False
Descriptive of musculoskeletal pain.

273. False
Suggestive of aortic dissection, massive pulmonary embolism or pneumothorax.

274. False
A choking sensation is common in angina and described by patients as breathlessness.

275. True

276. False
Maintaining contact can be useful.

277. True

278. False
No allowance is given in most cases.

279. True

280. True

281. False
Progesterone sufficiency in the second half of the cycle.

282. False
Accuracy is whether the measured value is close to the true value. Precision is the ability to detect small fluctuations in the measurements. The basal body temperature chart documents small changes daily and thus precision is more important than accuracy. Electronic thermometers may be less accurate but more precise than mercury thermometers and thus should be used in preference.

283. True

284. False
Early first intercourse.

285. False
Partner with genital warts or HPV infection of the genitals.

286. False
Being dark-skinned is a risk factor.

287. True
Caused by HPV, thus increasing the risk.

288. True

289. False
Women.

290. **True**

291. **True**

292. **True**

293. **True**

294. **False**
A sign, not a symptom.

295. **True**
In torsion, rupture or haemorrhage.

296. **False**
A sign.

297. **True**
For hormone-secreting tumours.

298. **True**

299. **True**

300. **True**

301. **False**
About 5% for all types of abuse.

302. **True**

303. **True**

304. **True**

305. **True**

306. **False**
Inadequate to cover *Haemophilus influenzae*. Amoxycillin, a beta-lactam plus beta-lactamase inhibitor combination, or a second-generation cephalosporin is better.

307. **True**
In cases related to dental procedures, where anaerobes are prevalent.

308. **False**
Cheek swelling should suggest either dental problems or maxillary carcinoma.

309. **False**
Altered colour or texture.

310. **True**

311. **False**
This is a nodule.

312. **False**
This is an abscess.

313. **False**
This is a petechiae.

314. **False**
Squamous epithelium is replaced with columnar epithelium.

315. True

But postcoital bleeding must not be assumed to be caused by ectropion. Full examination and possibly investigation are needed.

316. False

An excess of secreting glands.

317. False

Ectropion means cervical erosion.

318. True

319. True

Increases the intra-abdominal pressure.

320. True

This reduces the LOS pressure and impairs mucosal protection.

321. True

This relaxes the LOS.

322. True

Increases the intra-abdominal pressure and relaxes the LOS.

323. True

Relaxes the LOS and impairs mucosal protection.

324. False

325. True

326. True

327. False

328. False

329. False

Sensory loss on dorsal aspect of thumb only.

330. False

Sensory loss on lateral palm, thumb, index finger, middle finger and lateral aspect of ring finger.

331. False

Weakness of dorsiflexsion and eversion of foot.

332. True

333. False

Weakness of supinator.

334. True

335. True

336. False

Cogwheel or leadpipe rigidity is characteristic of extrapyramidal disorders. Clasp-knife rigidity suggests upper motor neuron lesion.

337. False

Worse at rest.

237

338. True

339. K

Normal chest findings do not rule out a pneumothorax.

340. H

The sinus bradycardia is caused by vagal stimulation in inferior infarction.

341. G

342. J

She has pneumonia with pleuritis. Pleural rub is not always present. When present it is easily missed.

343. D

Oesophageal pain is commonly relieved by nitrates.

344. A

345. F

The physical finding is incompatible with the history. The history of congenital heart disease is flawed. The ECG belongs to someone else.

346. D

The presence of epicanthic folds does not exclude a real manifest ocular squint.

347. L

348. K

With few exceptions, diplopia means paralytic squint.

349. H

350. J

351. K

352. D

353. B

354. C

Index

Index

Index

Prescribing, 220
  antibiotics, 124
Professional misconduct, 153
Pruritus ani, 126
Psoriasis, 187, 215
Puberty
  age of, 134
  delayed, 119–120

R
Rabies, 127
Ramsay Hunt syndrome, 212
Rape, 67–69
Rashes, 193
  childhood, 65–66
Records *see* Medical records
Red eye(s), 162–163
Reflux oesophagitis, 130, 220
Respiratory tract infections
  antibiotics, 160
  viral, causal associations, 182
Retinopathy, hypertensive, 124
Retirement, 59–60
Rheumatoid hand, 128
Rhinitis
  allergic, 159, 188
  vasomotor, 123
Rinne's test, 130
Roseola infantum, 65–66
Rotator cuff lesions, 131
Rubella, 129

S
Safety, place of (National Assistance Act),
  159
Salivary glands
  calculi, 152
  tumours, 191
Salmonellosis, 153
Salpingitis, 155, 189
Scabies, 43–44
Scaphoid, fractured, 128
Schizophrenia, first rank symptoms, 151
School health service, 188
Scoliosis
  idiopathic adolescent, 49–51
  Wilson and Jungner's criteria, 51
Screening
  antenatal, 97–99
  cervical smear programme, 126
Screening tests
  criteria, 151
  UK, 183
Second referral, request for, 15–16
Self-harm, risk, 36–37
Semen analysis, 127

Sex education, Education Act (1986), 161
Sexually transmitted diseases (STDs), 34v35
  genital herpes, 100–101
  rape cases, 68
  travel and, 71–72
  viral hepatitis, 125
Shoulder
  dislocation
    anterior, 190
    posterior, 125
    recurrent, 210
  frozen, 123
Sinus rhythms, 160
Sinusitis
  acute frontal, 128
  acute maxillary, 219
Skin abscesses, intravenous drug addict,
  87–88
Skin lesions, 219
  scaly, 156
Sleep apnoea syndrome, 183
Social phobia, 113–114
Spondylosis, cervical, 82, 217
Squint, 221–222
Staff, practice, treatment of, 64
Stillbirth rate, 214
Stones *see* Calculi
Stridor, 30-month-old child, 130
Stroke
  function loss following, 117–118
  possible effects on partner, 118
Substance abuse, 127, 214
Suicide, 154, 36–37

T
Temper tantrums, 74
Temperature chart, basal body temperature,
  218
Temporal lobe abscess, right, 218
Tennis elbow, 41–42, 155
Tetanus immunisation, 46
Tetracyclines, 184
Thiazides, 131
Thioridazine, adverse effects, 20
Throat, sore, bacterial/viral distinction, 158
Tinnitus, 216
Tonsils, abscess, 183
Torticollis, infantile, 184
Tracheostomy, emergency, 128
Travel to India, 70–72
Trichimonas vaginalis infestation, 158
Tuning fork tests, 157

U
Urethral caruncle, 130
Urinary tract infections, recurrent, 157